7 YEARS YOUNGER

THE ANTI-AGING BREAKTHROUGH

DIET

WORKBOOK

BY THE EDITORS OF GOOD HOUSEKEEPING

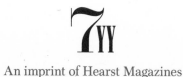

7YY

An imprint of Hearst Magazines

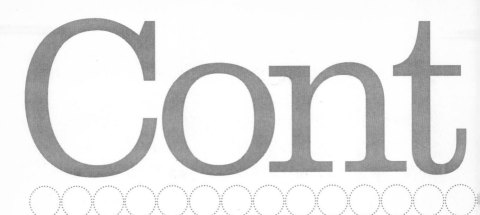

Cont

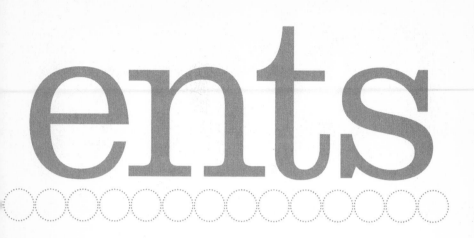

PART II
And Away You Go!

INTRODUCTION

Meet Your New Best Friend

I f you had a personal trainer—that is, someone to help you stay motivated and on track—would it help you attain the slimmer, younger-looking body you've been dreaming of? If the answer is yes, you're in luck. Let us introduce you to your new support system: You! With the 7 *Years Younger Anti-Aging Breakthrough Diet Workbook*, you'll have the power to identify your eating triggers, monitor your progress, and find ways to set new, healthier patterns. Your "trainer" will be there to provide a safe sounding board for the emotions that lead to overeating and to help you learn from your setbacks and celebrate your successes. You'll get daily guidance and feedback—just as if you had a real coach on call.

How does it work? Like a diary, this workbook allows you to commit your actions, thoughts, and feelings to paper. That alone can give you a clearer picture of how you're doing and help you recognize eating triggers. But unlike a diary, this workbook also speaks to you. Each day it gives you anti-aging advice, encouragement, and food for thought. On one day, for instance, you may find tips on quieting your food cravings and consuming fewer calories when you dine out; the following day, you'll see advice on kicking up your activity level and getting a handle on stress eating. We'll also share pointers from some of the best experts on weight loss we know—dieters who've shed pounds themselves.

This workbook is designed to be a companion to the 7 *Years Younger Anti-Aging Breakthrough Diet* and to help you get the most from that groundbreaking program. By combining reliable weight-loss strategies with advances in anti-aging science and introducing you to anti-aging foods, the 7 *Years Younger Anti-Aging Breakthrough Diet* doubles your results: Not only will you flatten your belly and slim your hips, but you'll diminish the lines on your face, too. Plus, y have a more energetic spring in your step, skin that glows, a lower risk of conditions like cancer and heart disease, and a reduced likelihood of mental decline or age-related maladies. With no special gimmicks on our part or any Herculean effort on yours—in fact, the program is fun and easy to follow—the *7 Years Younger Anti-Aging Breakthrough Diet* rejuvenates your health, restores your energy, and gives you a leaner body...in just seven weeks!

That's a statement we can make with confidence because, in the time-honored *Good Housekeeping* tradition, we put the diet to the test. Our intrepid panel of 26 men and women, ranging in age from 34 to 62, were given the same food plan, the same recipes, and the same recommendations for turning healthy eating into a lifestyle as those outlined in the *7 Years Younger Anti-Aging Breakthrough Diet.* When the seven weeks were up, they'd collectively lost 325 pounds and 105 inches. Two women lost as much as 19 pounds; one lost 9¼ inches around the waist! One male tester shed 23 pounds and 5½ inches, and another lost 28 pounds. The entire panel had remarkable results. The proof was in.

So, as it turned out, were the insights into what really helps people stick to a program and make lasting changes in their lives. Which brings us to what this workbook is all about: All of the *7 Years Younger Anti-Aging Breakthrough Diet* testers kept a journal during their time on the program, and many of them cited it as a major factor in their success. "Keeping the diary showed me how much sugar I was eating throughout the day," said Elizabeth Worthy, 43, an events manager, whose journal revealed just how much soda she was drinking: "Just giving that up probably played a key role in my losing 11 pounds in seven weeks." Malaika Adero, a 56-year-old editor, reported that keeping a journal did more than help her achieve her 8-pound loss. "It teaches you so much about how much food you really eat," she says. "I found out that eating well means eating quality food in the right quantity."

Our testers' experience is right in line with what research reveals about the benefits of keeping a journal when you're trying to shed pounds. In fact, the difference between results for those who keep a diet log and for those who do not keep one is remarkable. In 2008, researchers followed 1,700 men and women as they tried to lose weight by cutting back on calories and engaging in moderate-intensity physical activity. The study participants were asked to keep food records, too. At the end of six months, those who'd adhered to the journal-keeping request lost twice as much—an average of 18 pounds—as those who'd opted not to keep records. And the more conscientious the dieters were about recording their meals, the more weight they lost. The same was true of women who took part in a yearlong study at the Fred Hutchinson Cancer Research Center in Seattle in 2012. All of the 123 participating women were encouraged to record their food intake. Those who were more diligent about record-keeping lost close to 4% more than the less frequent journalers.

THE WRITE STUFF
Why does journal-keeping work so well for dieters?

One reason is that it helps clue you in to eating behaviors you may not even be aware of. Some ways in which you undermine your health will be obvious, of course. For instance, eating a lot of fast food and indulging your sweet tooth with big portions of cookies and ice cream are known to increase the risk of obesity and disease—if you know that's what you're doing. Sometimes habits are so ingrained, we don't even notice them. And there are lots of little ways to take in calories that can easily slip under your radar. How many times have you finished the leftovers on your kids' plates while clearing the dinner table, grabbed a handful of M&M's from the candy dish on a coworker's desk, or added another shake from the cereal box to your bowl to soak up leftover milk, barely giving it a thought? It's easy to eat mindlessly, never even registering what you're doing—which is exactly why having to account for every morsel you consume can be so eye-opening. Suddenly, all those bites that "didn't count" are in black and white on the page, where it's much harder to ignore them. As was true for our panelists, analyzing your eating patterns will likely open your eyes to the ways in which you've been sabotaging yourself without being aware of it.

Logging your food intake also makes you accountable to someone: yourself. Knowing that you'll later have to commit your dietary missteps to paper can make you think twice about choosing the fish and chips over the grilled halibut or taking that second helping. Even if you're the only one who's reading your f log, recognizing when you're going overboard gives you the tools to start to tackle those eating habits. On the flip side, being able to record a day when you stayed on track and met your goals will feel inspiring. Every time you scribble down the list of anti-aging foods in moderate portions that you ate, you'll reinforce just how capable you are of accomplishing what you put your mind to.

The workbook will also help you chronicle other important aspects of your day that relate to slimming down and looking younger. One of these is your hunger level. Eating only when you're truly hungry (and stopping before you're over-full) is key to weight loss and healthier living. Sometimes the urge to eat is just that—an urge, not a sign that your body really needs food. Being asked to record your hunger level before you eat can help you consider whether you're really following your appetite, just satisfying a craving, or eating because you're bored. It may even stop you in your tracks, helping you to avoid calories you don't really want or need.

A week's worth of hunger-level entries will also give you a good overview of your eating behavior. Are you relying on your body's true hunger cues, or are you eating for other reasons? And could one of those reasons be to ease emotional pain or anxiety? This workbook will help you find out. A bad day at work, a fight with your spouse or children, grieving, feeling lonely or underappreciated—they're all stressors that can lead to attempts to self-soothe, perhaps with diet-unfriendly foods like red velvet cupcakes and kettle-cooked chips. By creating space for you to write about your feelings, this workbook gives you the opportunity to make associations ("Feeling guilty about fight with Mom, downed a large candy bar") as well as a chance to work out some of those feelings on paper. According to Bruce Rabin, M.D., a professor of pathology and psychiatry at the University of Pittsburgh School of Medicine, writing about what's bothering you can create clarity and help reduce anxiety, lowering the likelihood of emotional eating.

Another aspect of your day you'll be documenting in this workbook is movement. Note that we've allotted space to record movement, not just formal workouts. There's little disagreement about how important exercise is for turning back the clock and maintaining weight loss—people who exercise regularly have fitter, younger-looking bodies; avoid some of the health hazards that come from sedentary living (among them high cholesterol, triglycerides, blood pressure, and blood sugar); and stay in better shape as they get older. Some researchers also believe that exercise may give you more willpower, making dieting easier. But as much as we encourage you to engage in formal workouts (the 7 *Years Younger Anti-Aging Breakthrough Diet* maps it out for you in a very simple way), we don't want you to discount any extra movement you do in a day. Climbing stairs, walking to the bus, hoofing it to the market three blocks away—it all counts! That's important because every time you jot down your daily activity, you're going to feel a wave of pride wash over you. We're willing to wager that recording your movement will motivate you to do even more.

THE 7 YEARS YOUNGER
ANTI-AGING BREAKTHROUGH
DIET BASICS

I f you haven't already checked out the 7 *Years Younger Anti-Aging Breakthrough Diet,* we think you'll be pleasantly surprised by how flexible and easy to follow it is. Because the diet is designed for simplicity and convenience, you can swap one breakfast for another and even the occasional lunch for a dinner (as long as you have an extra snack or eat a bit more with dinner so you don't get hungry). That means you're able to select the foods you like rather than being tied to a rigid menu. Good Housekeeping Research Institute Nutrition Director Samantha Cassetty, M.S., R.D., who designed and developed the diet, cleverly worked choice into it by creating a 3-4-5 Plan: All the breakfasts are around 300 calories; all the lunches, 400; and all the dinners, 500. Following a one-week Jumpstart, women can add in 250 calories' worth of snacks, and men, between 375 and 500 snack calories, depending on activity level. Plus, all the meals and snacks Sam has planned for you fit the calorie parameters, so you don't have to give the numbers a second thought.

In addition to having exceptional flexibility, this weight-loss plan was designed to provide delicious foods packed with nutrients that fight aging. It's particularly rich in antioxidants and omega-3 fatty acids, both shown to help prevent and diminish wrinkles, brighten skin, and reduce the kind of inflammation associated

Reclaim Your Good Health and Youth

E xperts believe that genetics plays a role in only about 25% of our risk of age-related illnesses. That means your lifestyle choices can make a huge difference in how healthy you are. And, as we've seen with the 7 *Years Younger Anti-Aging Breakthrough Diet* testers, those choices can make a significant difference in how youthful you look and how vibrant you feel, too. Every day on the diet will be helping you to:

- **Fight obesity and target belly fat,** the number one risk factor for heart disease, diabetes, stroke, and other life-threatening conditions

- **Fight chronic inflammation in the body,** which is believed to be at the root of many age-related diseases and health conditions

- **Protect your bones and keep them strong**

- **Reduce harmful LDL cholesterol and boost protective HDL cholesterol**

- **Normalize or lower blood pressure**

- **Regulate blood sugar levels and fight insulin resistance,** which can lead to type 2 diabetes

- **Protect against certain forms of cancer**

- **Help protect skin against the sun's harmful ultraviolet rays,** which cause wrinkles, age skin, and increase the risk of skin cancer

- **Nourish the skin and strengthen collagen,** the substance that keeps it supple and discourages wrinkles, frown lines, and jowls

- **Improve eye health**

with age-related health problems like arthritis and diabetes. Just shedding pounds can help you live longer and halt the age-accelerating effects of being overweight, but by losing weight the 7 Years Younger way, you're also fighting aging on the cellular level, ensuring that you end up looking both leaner and more youthful at the end of seven weeks. You'll be feeling more youthful, too: The *7 Years Younger Anti-Aging Breakthrough Diet* is like going to energy rehab; it recharges your engine.

One of the features of the plan that surprised many of our testers is that the diet doesn't leave you hungry. "I've found that eating this way, I am not hungry like I used to be, especially after exercising," says Leigh Gillam, 56, an office manager who lost 12 pounds in seven weeks on the diet. It's no accident: Knowing that many dieters typically give up because they're just too hungry, Sam carefully calibrated the diet in order to keep the calorie intake high enough to be filling, but low enough to facilitate weight loss. It's a delicate balance, but the 3-4-5 formula works.

Through the years, we at *Good Housekeeping* have talked to more than our share of men and women who've tried and failed to lose weight. Because of their feedback, we know a program that is overly complicated, leaves you hungry, or bores you to tears will fail faster than you can say "steamed vegetables." Fortunately, Sam and Susan Westmoreland, the GHRI food director, whose team developed and tested the 7 Years Younger dinner recipes, had the knowledge and expertise necessary to devise a plan that's simple to follow, filling, brimming with variety—it draws from various corners of the world, but especially from the never-dreary Mediterranean diet—and 100% delectable. "I honestly don't feel like I'm on a diet at all," said tester Maria Arap, 38, while on the road to her 10½-pound weight loss. "Honestly, for me, the hardest part is picking which recipe I want to make, because I like them all."

The 3-4-5 Plan is based on a wide-ranging array of colorful fruits and vegetables—they make up at least half the plate of every meal. It also calls for generous amounts of protein every day, primarily in the form of lean meats and poultry, seafood, legumes, and eggs. For variety, low-fat or fat-free dairy, tofu, and even whole grains add to the diet's protein content and round out the diet. The extra protein will help maintain your muscle mass, which tends to diminish with age and when you cut calories. Protein is also extremely satisfying, offering protection against hunger pangs every day, throughout the seven weeks.

At first (and maybe even second!) glance, the 7 Years Younger recipes don't look like diet dishes at all. Grilled Fish Tacos, Caprese Salad, Cold Peanut Noodles with Chicken, Pulled Pork on a Bun... you can see right away that you're not going to feel deprived. Perhaps even more surprising, you're not going to spend a lot of time in the kitchen. All of the recipes are easy to make, with prep times that usually come in at 30 minutes or less. Our menus also allow you to augment the diet with selected convenience foods, all of which have been vetted by the Good Housekeeping Research Institute to ensure that they're healthy and tasty and that they'll contribute to helping you get thinner and look younger.

As you record your food choices in this workbook, you'll be able to note favorite recipes and go-to snacks during the next seven weeks. On those days when you're wavering, perhaps tempted to return to old eating habits, a glance back at your log will remind you of all the nutritious and delicious options you have at your disposal. That's something you can do even after you've reached the end of the diet to help you maintain your new, slimmer body and continue to reap anti-aging benefits well beyond the plan's seven weeks. Think of it as a road map for the rest of your life.

Want to be a test panelist for a future 7 Years Younger plan?
Sign up at 7yearsyounger.com/panelist to be considered.

HOW TO USE THIS WORKBOOK

I f you've ever kept a journal before, you might have set aside one particular time of day to record the events and details of the previous 24 hours. We're asking you to check in more often than that to help you get the most accurate record of everything you consume during the day—and, just as important, your hunger level and emotional state. Before you eat, note your hunger level on a scale of 1 to 4 as follows: 1 = full; 2 = not hungry; 3 = hungry; 4 = very hungry. Being able to assess your feelings and actions will go a long way toward helping you understand—and change—any habits that stand in the way of your success.

The workbook provides you with writing space for each day of the 7 Years Younger Anti-Aging Breakthrough Diet (that's 49 days, if you're counting). There are some constants. Each day has a place for you to enter what you ate, how hungry you were, and the emotions you felt at the time. You'll also write down your exercise and other activities. In addition, weight-loss tips, fitness strategies, motivating advice, and anti-aging information appear throughout to help you stay on track.

HUNGER LEVEL
Before Eating

1 • Full

2 • Not hungry

3 • Hungry

4 • Very hungry

How much time should you spend on the workbook?

That's up to you, but the more detailed you get and the more you use the blank space as an outlet for your thoughts and feelings, the more you're going to get out of the journal. Here's what a typical day with your workbook might look like:

1 **Set aside a few minutes before breakfast** (or the night before) to take a look at the workbook. Read the to-do list and thumb through the day's pages for tips to help you throughout the next 24 hours (and beyond). Also go over the shopping lists: Do you have everything you need for the next few days? Is a trip to the grocery store in order? When you're ready to eat, assess your hunger level, jot it down, and enjoy one of the delicious 7 Years Younger breakfasts. Even though it's first thing in the morning, don't neglect the "Emotions" section. Perhaps you're feeling invigorated and optimistic as you begin your day. Maybe you're dreading going to work. Positive or negative, write it down!

2 **We encourage you to carry the workbook around with you** during the day, but if that's not possible, make sure you at least have a pen and paper at hand. (If you prefer an app for keeping track and for calorie counting, Sam recommends Lose It!) Then, any time you eat, record all the relevant information; you can copy it into your workbook in the evening. Be sure to write down any ordinary activity you do throughout the day—taking the stairs in a department store, walking to a park to eat lunch, trekking across a big parking lot. Get it all down—and see if you can do even more the next day.

3 **In the evening, after dinner or before bed,** spend some time going over your day. Fill in any exercise you participated in as well as the "Daily Assessment" section. Give yourself some time to really think about how the day went. Evaluate what went right, and learn from any slipups. For instance, if you missed eating a good breakfast in the morning, now's the time to think about why. Was it because you didn't get up early enough? Resolve to make a change (go to bed earlier, get a more insistent alarm clock) that will help you get at the root of the problem. In the end, whether your day went perfectly or not, congratulate yourself for being persistent. Taking the time to pay close attention to your day is a huge step in the direction of reaching your goals.

4 **Before you close the book, give some thought to tomorrow.** Plan your meals so you won't find yourself standing at a vending machine or fast-food counter because you didn't stop at the grocery store and you don't have a satisfying snack or the fixings for one of the 7 Years Younger packable lunches. Consciously set your intentions for the day, and you'll be much more likely to stick to them.

7 YEARS YOUNGER RESOURCES TO HELP YOU STAY ON TRACK!

Free Stuff

- **Get our free weekly anti-aging newsletter** at 7yearsyounger.com/newsletter

Download our free anti-aging reports, filled with helpful, doable tips:

- **40 Best Anti-Aging Beauty Secrets** at 7yearsyounger.com/antiagingsecrets

- **Best Anti-Aging Makeup** at 7yearsyounger.com/makeup

- **Eat to Look and Feel Younger** at 7yearsyounger.com/eattolookyoung

- **50 Ways to Stress Less & Live Longer** at 7yearsyounger.com/stressless

Shopping

- **To find our top rated anti-aging beauty products,** visit 7yearsyounger.com/shop

- **To buy a copy of the *New York Times* best seller *7 Years Younger: The Revolutionary 7-Week Anti-Aging Plan,*** go to 7yearsyounger.com/book

- **To buy a copy of *7 Years Younger: The Anti-Aging Breakthrough Diet,*** go to 7yearsyounger.com/dietworkbook

- **Find out about the 7 Years Younger Plan from Nutrisystem** at nutrisystem.com/7yy

- **To get up-to-the-minute anti-aging health and diet news,** subscribe to *Good Housekeeping* at 7yy.goodhousekeeping.com

Social

- **Like us on facebook.com/7yearsyounger** and join us there for daily tips and inspiration

- **Follow us on Twitter** @7yearsyounger

- **Follow us on** pinterest.com/7yearsyounger

PART I

How To Prep for the Last Diet You'll Ever Need

MAKE A COMMITMENT

Purchasing a diet book, shopping for healthy foods, signing up for a gym membership—those are all ways to make a commitment to becoming thinner, healthier, and more youthful. But while putting your money where your mouth is can help you commit to change, it's just as important—maybe even more important—to make a formal promise to yourself. You can do that by writing it down, in effect creating a pact with yourself. When you see a commitment on paper, it can feel more real, and that can make it harder to renege on it.

To begin, think about your goals—and not just the large ones, like "I want to look as slim and young as I did before I had my first child," but also the small ones, such as "I'm going to get my bicycle out of the garage and ride it three times a week." Revisit your pledge often in order to stay focused on your goals and remind yourself of why you're making the effort. You can even use your pledge as a guide to visualizing a new you, a process that can help make aspirations become realities. At McGill University in Montreal, for instance, researchers had people write down a pledge to eat more fruit, then picture themselves buying and preparing it. The combination of visualization and writing down their healthy promise led them to eat twice as much fruit as people who simply vowed to include more of it in their diets.

You'll find a sample pledge on page 18. You can adopt this pledge as is or use it as a template to create your own unique version.

I dedicate the next seven weeks to following the *7 Years Younger Anti-Aging Breakthrough Diet* program.

My goal is to look and feel the very best that I possibly can.

I will invest the time and energy needed to follow the program.

I know that there will be challenging moments along the way, but with each new day I have another chance to continue the transformation that I have promised myself.

I will look to my family and friends to support me during these seven weeks and beyond, and I will support others making the same journey.

I am grateful for this opportunity to improve myself and to bring lasting positive changes into my life.

_____ Day of _____ 20_____

_____
(Signature)

PLEDGES FROM OUR PANELISTS

The following are a few of the pledges our panelists wrote, meant to inspire you to craft one that's uniquely your own. Writing a pledge tailored to your own needs will make the process more meaningful to you and allow you to address any specific issues you may be struggling with.

1 Fewer Calories, More Enjoyment

- I pledge to spend the next seven weeks rolling back the past seven years of my life.
- By sticking to the 7 *Years Younger Anti-Aging Breakthrough Diet* plan, I propose to finally implement calorie control, breaking habits of overeating and emotional eating that have dominated my weight throughout my adult life.
- I pledge to use the food journal—I'm understandably scared, as it will be my first experience with this weight-loss tool—to help me finally gain control over food, which has for too long held the upper hand with me. I commit to chronicling each meal, snack, and drink, and to treating myself lovingly, to being honest about any daily shortcomings while still pushing myself to finally eat to live, a contrast to all the years I've spent living to eat.
- I pledge to celebrate and enjoy this time of discipline, self-control, health, and wellness as the foundation of a future lifetime of eating healthfully, having a solid, healthy relationship with food, enjoying exercise, and becoming the person I've always wanted to be.
- And I pledge to remain grateful for this amazing opportunity each and every day.

2 Heading Diabetes Off at the Pass

- I am embarking on this journey to lose weight, look better, and feel better about myself. I realize that sticking to the diet and exercise requirements will be challenging, but I will make every effort to change my lifestyle to live a longer and healthier life. I am doing this along with my wonderful wife to show support for her participation in this program and to help her meet her goals.

- Losing at least 10 pounds will also help me to avoid developing diabetes, which runs in my family. I am looking forward to achieving a mental and physical transformation that will benefit me for the rest of my life.

3 Tapping Into Support

- I pledge to put as much effort into this program as the experts have put into designing it. I will follow the program so that results published in the future will be as honest as possible.
- I pledge not to cheat myself of expert advice and opinions and to take full advantage of the unique opportunity given to me.
- I pledge to use my support system to help maximize results and motivate me. This includes family and friends as well as professionals at my gym and other panelists and professionals through whatever means are offered as part of this program.
- I pledge to offer "real life" results—i.e., when truly special events and/ or overwhelming temptation causes a hiccup in my efforts, I'll get right back on the plan.
- I pledge to get back into the pool again, which I truly enjoy and haven't been doing.

4 No Whining!

- I am going to enjoy this.
- Maybe not every minute or every second, and there will surely be times when I want to quit. But I will enjoy it because I'm doing something good—very good—for myself.
- I am committed to doing whatever is required during the coming weeks to complete the 7 *Years Younger Anti-Aging Breakthrough Diet* challenge.
- Bottom line: I want to feel—and look—as good as I can. If I begin to "whine" about having less wine—or no ice cream—or not having a second bowl of brown rice (sadly, just because it's brown rice doesn't mean you can eat as much as you want!), maybe I can stop and focus

instead on how lucky I am to be in this program.

- And one more bottom line: I spend too much time worrying about others and not enough time doing what it takes to give myself the best life possible. This is an opportunity to turn that around.
- I pledge to remind myself what a joy that will be—to focus on me! And I'll keep reminding myself until it sticks!

IT TAKES A VILLAGE (OR AT LEAST A BUDDY)

Ultimately, the results you get from this program will depend on your actions. But no dieter need be completely on his or her own. Having the support of friends and family can go a long way toward helping you reach your goals. You can harness the help of others by not only telling trusted allies your plans for the next seven weeks, but also explaining how they can assist you. Make a list of what you need to help guide you in making your request. Maybe it's help from a friend who can give you shopping and cooking advice. Maybe it's for your family to be understanding and accepting while you restock the cupboards and rule the menu for the weeks to come. Or maybe you just need someone who can talk you down from the step stool as you reach into the cookie cupboard. Also target times of the day when you'll need support: Could a call from a friend who gets up early help you hit the treadmill in the morning? Be strategic in your planning.

If you can take it a step further and have a friend or family member buddy up with you on the *7 Years Younger Anti-Aging Breakthrough Diet,* or even just for exercise, all the better. Research has shown that dieters who have a partner are more likely to stick with their plans than those who go it alone, and that they lose more weight. And it's not just because they share recipes or work out together. Co-dieters connect psychologically. They empathize with, commiserate with, and encourage each other, and they celebrate together. There were several couples among our panelists, and they told us that doing the program together was extremely helpful. "Going on the diet with a partner—in my case, my husband—made it much easier to do the shopping and removed the temptation of eating fattening foods that otherwise find their way into the kitchen when only one person in the household is dieting," says Michele Fredman, 61, a lawyer who lost 7½ pounds.

Connecting with a wider community can be useful, too. Throughout the seven weeks on the program, our diet testers kept in touch on Facebook. They chatted, exchanged tips, and cheered one another on. (You can check us out on facebook .com/7yearsyounger and join us there for daily tips and inspiration.) Similarly, there are many interactive weight-loss websites, including our own 7yearsyounger .com as well as sparkpeople.com. Connecting online has been shown to help keep lost pounds from returning. A study at Kaiser Permanente followed 348 successful dieters and found that those who logged on to a diet-and-fitness website at least once a month for two and a half years kept off more pounds than those who stopped connecting (or visited the sites less often).

SETTING A WEIGHT-LOSS GOAL

So many variables govern well-being that experts have struggled to come up with a way of ascertaining how much any specific person should weigh for optimum health. One measure commonly used for setting weight-loss goals is the Body Mass Index (BMI) formula, which uses height and weight to estimate body fat. It's imperfect—it may, for instance, overestimate body fat in people with muscular builds—but it can still give you a number to shoot for. The easiest way to determine your BMI is to plug your height and weight into an online calculator (ours is at goodhousekeeping.com/health /bmi-calculator). Here are the numbers that correspond with various weight levels:

Underweight = <18.5
Normal weight = 18.5-24.9
Overweight = 25-29.9
Obese = >30

Another measurement that's useful for goal-setting is waist circumference. We always measure the waistline of each of our diet testers because it's such an important indicator of health: The more fat you carry around your waist, the greater your risk of heart disease, hypertension, and diabetes. If you're a man with a 40-inch or larger waist circumference or a woman with a 35-inch or larger waist, you could be in the danger zone. To measure your own waist, place a tape measure around your middle, just above your hipbones, while standing. Measure after you breathe out. Then, to assess your risk, go to the NIH's website on healthy weight: nhlbi.nih.gov/health/public/heart/obesity /lose_wt/bmi_dis.htm.

Use your BMI and waist-circumference figures to gauge your starting point and set your sights on how far you'd like to go. You may drop anywhere from 10 to 25 pounds on the seven-week *7 Years Younger Anti-Aging Breakthrough Diet*—your results will depend on how much activity you do, how closely you stick to the plan, and, of course, your body's own unique biology. Depending on your goal, reaching it may mean sticking to the meal plans—or at least the same calorie levels—for more than seven weeks. (See page 271 for information on how to maintain your weight loss.)

When Sam created the diet's meal plan, she set the calorie counts at levels that are healthy and satisfying, but low enough to melt off pounds:

- **1,450 calories for women;**
- **1,575 calories for slightly to moderately active men** (which includes most men);
- **1,700 calories for highly active men** (meaning those who have labor-intensive jobs or who work out a good hour a day about five times a week).

How quickly will you lose? That depends. Most people lose both water weight and fat at the start of any diet, and that can skew the early results. As a general rule, you can expect to lose at least a pound a week, predicated on the idea that one pound of fat equals 3,500 calories. There are individual differences among dieters, but, for the most part, using the 3,500-calorie guideline will give you a pretty good sense of how quickly the pounds will drop off.

As you go through the next seven weeks, don't be discouraged if you aren't shedding pounds as quickly as you had hoped. Your body is unique! Honor it and keep your goals within a realistic realm. Stay positive, hit your daily calorie targets, and the results you want will come.

Daily Calorie Targets

For Women

Breakfast	300
Lunch	400
Dinner	500
Snacks (2)	250 *(total)*
TOTAL	**1,450**

For Men

Breakfast	300
Lunch	400
Dinner	500
Snacks (2)	375–500 *(total)*
TOTAL	**1,575–1,700**

WHAT KIND OF EATER ARE YOU?

The aim of this workbook is to help you understand yourself better. Most of us know when we're ignoring the big healthy-eating guidelines ("Don't eat junk food," "Drive past the drive-through"), but we sometimes don't realize just how frequently we're flouting the rules. And sometimes we don't see our destructive patterns at all. This quiz is designed to help you zero in on your eating style. Use your score to determine your personal diet pitfalls so you can go about changing them. That's what the next seven weeks are all about.

1. When I'm hungry, fast food is an easy fix; I often stop and grab something—french fries, a burger, maybe a donut.
- **A.** Rarely *(0 points)*
- **B.** Sometimes *(1 point)*
- **C.** Often *(2 points)*
- **D.** Always *(3 points)*

2. While I never think about chips and never buy them, if they're in front of me (at a party or in the office break room, for example), I'll automatically snack on them.
- **A.** Rarely *(0 points)*
- **B.** Sometimes *(1 point)*
- **C.** Often *(2 points)*
- **D.** Always *(3 points)*

3. I'm usually not hungry in the morning, so I tend to run out of the house without eating breakfast.
- **A.** Rarely *(0 points)*
- **B.** Sometimes *(1 point)*
- **C.** Often *(2 points)*
- **D.** Always *(3 points)*

4. My hunger is often sudden and urgent, and, if I eat a large quantity of food, I feel guilty afterward.

A. Rarely *(0 points)*

B. Sometimes *(1 point)*

C. Often *(2 points)*

D. Always *(3 points)*

5. I drink juice, regular soda, or other sugary drinks a few times every day.

A. Rarely *(0 points)*

B. Sometimes *(1 point)*

C. Often *(2 points)*

D. Always *(3 points)*

6. I drink "sports" or "health" beverages like the regular versions of Gatorade and Vitaminwater.

A. Rarely *(0 points)*

B. Sometimes *(1 point)*

C. Often *(2 points)*

D. Always *(3 points)*

7. When I'm upset, I can eat a whole pizza (or a box of cookies, or a carton of ice cream) in one sitting and still want more.

A. Rarely *(0 points)*

B. Sometimes *(1 point)*

C. Often *(2 points)*

D. Always *(3 points)*

8. On very busy days, I may eat just one or two times a day.

A. Rarely *(0 points)*

B. Sometimes *(1 point)*

C. Often *(2 points)*

D. Always *(3 points)*

9. I tend to nibble on whatever foods my family or friends don't finish, even when I'm full.
- **A.** Rarely *(0 points)*
- **B.** Sometimes *(1 point)*
- **C.** Often *(2 points)*
- **D.** Always *(3 points)*

10. Low-fat pastries and muffins and sugar-free sweets and cookies are my diet go-tos.
- **A.** Rarely *(0 points)*
- **B.** Sometimes *(1 point)*
- **C.** Often *(2 points)*
- **D.** Always *(3 points)*

11. The vegetables most often on my plate are french fries.
- **A.** Rarely *(0 points)*
- **B.** Sometimes *(1 point)*
- **C.** Often *(2 points)*
- **D.** Always *(3 points)*

12. While cooking or preparing food, I tend to taste it so many times that I'm not really hungry when I finally sit down to eat the meal.
- **A.** Rarely *(0 points)*
- **B.** Sometimes *(1 point)*
- **C.** Often *(2 points)*
- **D.** Always *(3 points)*

13. At a certain time of day, I find myself ravenous and searching for something to quiet my growling stomach.
- **A.** Rarely *(0 points)*
- **B.** Sometimes *(1 point)*
- **C.** Often *(2 points)*
- **D.** Always *(3 points)*

14. After a stressful day, food provides a welcome distraction from my anxious feelings.

    A. Rarely *(0 points)*

    B. Sometimes *(1 point)*

    C. Often *(2 points)*

    D. Always *(3 points)*

15. I hit the drive-through a few times a week.

    A. Rarely *(0 points)*

    B. Sometimes *(1 point)*

    C. Often *(2 points)*

    D. Always *(3 points)*

16. I have at least two beers, glasses of wine, or other alcoholic drinks four or more times a week.

    A. Rarely *(0 points)*

    B. Sometimes *(1 point)*

    C. Often *(2 points)*

    D. Always *(3 points)*

17. While watching TV or a movie, I automatically reach for snacks, regardless of whether or not I'm hungry.

    A. Rarely *(0 points)*

    B. Sometimes *(1 point)*

    C. Often *(2 points)*

    D. Always *(3 points)*

18. Since I'm never sure where and when I'll have a real meal, I tend to eat on the fly.

    A. Rarely *(0 points)*

    B. Sometimes *(1 point)*

    C. Often *(2 points)*

    D. Always *(3 points)*

19. A bad day at work, a fight with a friend, or a family argument can trigger a binge.

    A. Rarely *(0 points)*

    B. Sometimes *(1 point)*

    C. Often *(2 points)*

    D. Always *(3 points)*

20. I have several cups of coffee or tea with sugar and/or cream or milk every day.

    A. Rarely *(0 points)*

    B. Sometimes *(1 point)*

    C. Often *(2 points)*

    D. Always *(3 points)*

TALLY 'EM UP

Use your answers to see which eating group—or groups (don't be surprised if you land in more than one)—you fall into. A score of six or more puts you squarely into the category. Use the awareness of your trouble spots to guide you as you go through the next seven weeks. Pay particular attention to tips that target those eating behaviors, and document your progress each week.

Junk Food Junkie score:

Add points from questions 1, 10, 11, and 15: _____

Junk Food Junkies fill up on nutrient-poor (empty-calorie) foods. Fast foods, sugary snacks, salty munchies, and high-fat fare are the norm; vegetables, fruits, whole grains, and other healthy picks are less frequent choices.

Mindless Muncher score:

Add points from questions 2, 9, 12, and 17: _____

Mindless Munchers are all-day grazers and unconscious eaters who put food in their mouths out of habit or boredom, regardless of hunger. They'll eat in front of the TV or automatically snack at a party, for example, paying little attention to their hunger cues. When Mindless Munchers start to track what they consume, they're often surprised at how much they eat during the course of the day.

Meal Skipper score:

Add points from questions 3, 8, 13, and 18: _____

Meal Skippers tend to have unbalanced eating patterns and often wait too long between meals. As a result, their meals are not planned or thought out, but rather are last-minute choices made wherever and whenever hunger takes over. They often end up making poor diet choices and caving in to cravings because they're so famished.

Emotional Eater score:

Add points from questions 4, 7, 14, and 19: _____

Emotional Eaters use food for more than fuel—it also serves as a friend and a comfort. Feelings such as sadness, loneliness, anger, boredom, and frustration cause these eaters to turn to food for escape.

Liquid-Calorie Lover score:

Add points from questions 5, 6, 16, and 20: _____

Liquid-Calorie Lovers unwittingly load their diets with extra calories from drinks. Sodas, milkshakes, coffee drinks, cocktails, smoothies, sports drinks, and more spell trouble for their caloric bottom line.

FIVE WEIGHT-LOSS AND ANTI-AGING STRATEGIES

A good meal plan, like the one Sam developed for the 7 *Years Younger Anti-Aging Breakthrough Diet,* goes a long way toward helping you shed pounds. When food is satisfying and nutrient-packed, yet calories are moderate, you've got a winning ticket to a thinner, younger-looking you. So don't let old habits and ingrained behaviors get in the way of letting this meal plan work its magic. You'll find tips and tricks threaded throughout these pages to help you move more, plan better, overcome cravings, and find alternatives to stress eating. The following five basic diet success principles can help you, too.

1 **Make your new lifestyle a priority** You undoubtedly have many responsibilities that demand your attention. Put losing weight and turning back the clock at the top of the list. Say no to coworkers who want you to go out for a drink after work when you know the happy-hour food will tempt you (suggest a walk instead). Schedule exercise and show up for it, just as you would for a doctor's appointment. Get up 10 minutes early and make your lunch so that you won't be consigned to the employee canteen's greatest fattening hits. Take the time to write in this workbook each day. While you would never let down another person who depended on you, it's all too easy to let your own needs fall by the wayside. Not this time. Make reaching your weight-loss and anti-aging goals your number one priority.

2 **Think about food in a new way** Calories are important, and your calorie intake is going to be what largely determines whether you blast off pounds or they stay put. However, it's also important to think beyond calories. Aim to eat foods that are nutrient-dense—that is, packed with vitamins, minerals, fiber, phytonutrients, and the other components that will make you look, feel, and, health-wise, essentially *be* younger. Nutrient-dense foods—versus those like french fries, chips, soda, and cookies that provide essentially empty calories—are the secret to losing weight and rejuvenating your skin and health. So be a food detective and scout out both nutrition facts and calories. Read food labels, gather nutrition brochures from your favorite dining spots, and go online and read food manufacturers' and restaurants' health stats. Check out the USDA's National Nutrient Database at ndb.nal.usda.gov for information on basic foods like cheeses and meats.

3 **Be a more mindful eater** Who says you're not paying attention to what you eat? You're preoccupied with food—that's the problem! Constantly thinking about your next meal is different than paying close attention to how and when you eat and how hungry you really are. Research shows that people who monitor their hunger level closely so they eat only when they truly need to and stop before they've overeaten maintain healthier weights. Likewise, experiencing your food as you eat it rather than gulping it down or being distracted by television or books can lead to a slimmer body. Mindfulness, the concept of being aware of the present moment, is a theme that runs through the 7 *Years Younger Anti-Aging Breakthrough Diet*. Use the how-tos throughout this workbook to help you develop new, more conscious (and more conscientious) eating habits.

4 **Start moving** Of the many misconceptions about exercise, one is that you must work out hard (i.e., be a sweating, panting mess on a daily basis) to gain any weight-loss benefit. That's not true. You can burn plenty of calories by simply walking, getting in several short bouts a day if you don't have the time to commit to a long session. What is true, though, is that you have to do *something* if you want to maintain weight loss and get the anti-aging benefits of this program. A sedentary lifestyle doesn't just thwart efforts to turn back the clock; it also accelerates the aging process. In addition, being sedentary makes it difficult to get pounds to budge—multiple studies show that dieters are vastly more successful when they both reduce calories and increase physical activity. If you're a late bloomer when it comes to exercise or need help restarting your workouts, the *7 Years Younger Anti-Aging Breakthrough Diet* has a comprehensive plan to help you. A good place to begin: Start incorporating more movement into your daily routine (see the tips scattered throughout this workbook).

5 **Believe in yourself** Success isn't a synonym for perfection. There will be hiccups along the way to reaching your weight and anti-aging goals; don't let them make you give up. Focus on all that you are accomplishing, and congratulate yourself along the way. Let each little triumph—making it through a movie without your usual vat of "butter"-soaked theater popcorn, spending half an hour of your lunch break going for a walk—be a reminder that you are capable of keeping your word to yourself. Remember, too, that all those day-to-day victories will add up to the big results you are dreaming of.

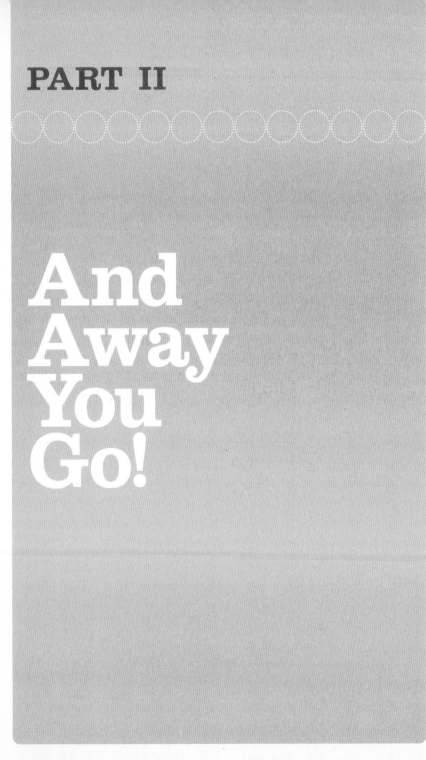

PART II

And Away You Go!

New beginnings are exciting, and this diet is no exception. It's going to give you a sense of renewal right out of the gate, and you're going to have fun exploring new ideas for cooking and eating. What's more, the magic isn't going to wear off after a week or two. The 7 *Years Younger Anti-Aging Breakthrough Diet* is designed to stay interesting the whole way through, then guide you into making the transition to eating healthfully and happily for a lifetime.

What follows is the plan's core shopping list. It's full of the pantry/refrigerator/freezer staples you'll need for the weeks to come, which will also serve you well once you've completed the seven-week plan. By giving your kitchen a makeover, you'll be giving your body a makeover, too.

To begin the diet, stock up on the items listed on the core shopping list and the items listed on the Week 1/Jumpstart list. At the end of each week, read ahead to the following week's shopping list so that you'll never be caught unprepared. Don't give yourself any excuses to deviate from the diet.

THE 7 YEARS YOUNGER ANTI-AGING BREAKTHROUGH DIET CORE SHOPPING LIST

With seven weeks' worth of menus, the *7 Years Younger Anti-Aging Breakthrough Diet* packs a lot of variety. We have made sure your taste buds won't tire of foods or flavors and that there's something for everyone and every craving. We've also taken the hassle out of grocery shopping by providing week-by-week lists that itemize the exact amount of food you'll need to prepare each of the recipes on that week's menu. If 2 tablespoons of soy sauce are needed for lunch one day and another 2 tablespoons are used for dinner two days later, you'll see that calculated as 4 tablespoons of soy sauce on the shopping list. You'll undoubtedly already have some of the ingredients on each list in your fridge, freezer, and pantry (especially as the weeks go on). By laying it all out, these shopping lists will help you decide whether you have what you need to cover your menu or you need to stock up.

In some cases, you may find that you don't have to follow the recipes (and, by extension, the shopping lists) to the letter. For instance, if breakfast includes low-sugar apricot preserves one day and a dessert calls for low-sugar raspberry preserves a few days later, you may prefer to buy just one or the other. There's also no need to spend extra cash buying three varieties of cheese slices or sticks—if you like Cheddar better than Swiss, buy that and stay with it. We will be including all ingredients on the shopping list, but we encourage you to make commonsense substitutions based on what you like, need, or already have on hand. So if a salad calls for arugula and you have leftover romaine lettuce, or a recipe calls for feta and you have an opened container of reduced-fat feta crumbles, save yourself the hassle of an extra trip to the market. Ingredient swaps are fine as long as you follow one rule of thumb: When making substitutions, always go for the lower-calorie option (i.e., the reduced-fat or low-fat version instead of the regular kind) to keep your weight loss on track.

NUTS, SEEDS & LEGUMES

Whole roasted unsalted almonds
Slivered or sliced almonds
Creamy no-sugar-added peanut butter
Walnut halves
Pine nuts
Pistachios
Pecans
Unsalted dry-roasted peanuts
Seapoint Farms Dry Roasted
  Edamame, Lightly Salted
  or Wasabi flavor
Sesame seeds

CEREALS & GRAINS

Multi Grain Cheerios
Plain instant oatmeal
Quick-cooking brown rice
Old-fashioned oats
Quick-cooking barley
Whole wheat bread crumbs
Bulgur

DAIRY

Plain fat-free yogurt
Plain nonfat Greek yogurt
Part-skim ricotta cheese
Large eggs
Pecorino Romano cheese
Parmesan cheese
Low-fat (1%) or fat-free milk
Reduced-fat cream cheese

SALAD DRESSINGS & CONDIMENTS

Reduced-fat ranch dressing
Reduced-fat balsamic vinegar dressing
Reduced-fat Caesar dressing
Chipotle sauce or other hot sauce
Spicy brown mustard
Dijon mustard
Light mayonnaise
Sun-dried tomatoes (not oil-packed)
Large black olives
Stir-fry sauce
Barbecue sauce
  (preferably no-sugar-added)
Reduced-sodium soy sauce
Horseradish mustard
Worcestershire sauce
Ketchup (fruit-sweetened, preferably
  with no sugar added)
Salsa
Anchovy paste (optional)
Sweet pickle relish

DRIED HERBS & SPICES

Smoked paprika
Salt-free chili powder
Dry mustard powder
Salt
Black pepper or peppercorns
Dried tarragon
Dried oregano
Cayenne pepper
Ground coriander
Ground cinnamon
Salt-free Cajun seasoning
Ground cumin
Crushed red pepper flakes
Curry powder
Dried dill
Garlic salt
Celery seeds
Ground allspice
Ancho chile powder

OILS & VINEGARS

Cooking spray
Olive oil
Canola oil
Vegetable oil
Apple cider vinegar
Balsamic vinegar
Asian sesame oil
White wine vinegar
Seasoned rice vinegar

BREAD*

Arnold Select 100% Whole Wheat
　Sandwich Thins
Whole-grain bread
Whole Wheat Thomas' Bagel Thins
La Tortilla Factory Smart & Delicious
　100% Whole Wheat Flatbread or
　whole-grain tortillas
Medium-size whole wheat pita breads
Whole-grain English muffins
1.5-ounce whole-grain rolls
Whole wheat hamburger buns
Corn tortillas
Whole-grain fruit/nut bread

FRESH PRODUCE

Lemons
Limes
Garlic
Red and yellow onions
Shallots
Fresh ginger

SPREADS

Low-sugar or no-sugar-added
　strawberry, peach, apricot, or
　grape preserves
100%-fruit orange marmalade
Margarine or butter

MISCELLANEOUS

Capers
Jarred roasted red peppers
Dry red wine
Dry white wine
Mini chocolate chips
Sugar-free pancake syrup
Dried plum bits or raisins
Dried figs
Brown sugar
Vanilla extract
Honey
Instant nonfat dry-milk powder
Dove Dark Chocolate Promises
Zero-calorie sweetener (optional)

*Store bread in the freezer so it will last
through the seven weeks. Refrigerate
tortillas. If you prefer to buy bread fresh
(or only have a small freezer), simply
purchase it weekly instead of considering
it a staple.

WEEK 1

Jumpstart

You're going to learn a lot about yourself this week. Writing about every bite you take, from the day's meals to that forkful of your spouse's chocolate cake, will reveal why you may be eating when you're not really hungry, the times when you're most vulnerable to overeating, and any unconscious munching you're engaging in. It's going to be enlightening and helpful in the weeks to come.

This week, your calorie intake will be slightly lower than in weeks two through seven: 1,200 a day for women; 1,450 for slightly to moderately active men; and 1,575 calories for very active men. The purpose is to get your weight loss into gear so you feel motivated to continue. Remember, too, that this book is full of helpful strategies.

WEEK 1

DAY 1
Breakfast: California Breakfast Bruschetta
Lunch: Chipotle Lunch
Dinner: Big Fusilli Bowl

DAY 2
Breakfast: Sweet Stuffed Waffle
Lunch: Garden Turkey Sandwich with Lemon Mayo
Dinner: Salmon with Peppers & Pilaf

DAY 3
Breakfast: New York Bagel
Lunch: Caprese Salad
Dinner: Steak & Oven Fries

DAY 4
Breakfast: Banana–Peanut Butter Smoothie
Lunch: Ham & Swiss
Dinner: Grilled Fish Tacos

DAY 5
Breakfast: Easy Oatmeal
Lunch: Mediterranean Hummus "Pizza"
Dinner: Pulled Pork on a Bun

DAY 6
Breakfast: Smoked-Salmon Scrambled Eggs
Lunch: Finger Food
Dinner: Turkey-Feta Burgers

DAY 7
Breakfast: Strawberry Cereal
Lunch: Microwavable Pasta Meal
Dinner: Chicken & Veggie Stir-Fry

Shopping List

For breakfasts, lunches, and dinners serving anywhere from one to six. Check recipes to make adjustments depending on the number of people you are feeding.

FRESH PRODUCE

- 1 bunch basil
- 1 large bunch chives
- 1 bunch cilantro
- 1 bunch mint
- 5 green onions
- 2 pints (12 ounces each) grape tomatoes
- 1 plum tomato
- 5 regular tomatoes
- 3 cups shredded cabbage mix
- 1 head romaine lettuce
- 8 ounces baby spinach
- 1 package (9 ounces) microwave-in-bag spinach
- 12 ounces fresh broccoli florets
- 2 cups shredded carrots
- 1 bunch celery
- 2 ears corn
- 3 small bell peppers (red, orange, and yellow)
- 1 large yellow bell pepper
- 3 baking potatoes (1½ pounds total)
- 2 avocados
- 3 bananas
- 20 cherries
- 1 small bunch red seedless grapes
- 1 honeydew melon
- 1 kiwifruit
- 1 small orange
- ½ cup pineapple chunks
- 1 pint (12 ounces) strawberries
- ¼ small watermelon

SEAFOOD

- 4 skinless center-cut salmon fillets (1½ pounds total)
- 1 pound skinless tilapia fillets
- 6 ounces lox or thinly sliced smoked salmon

MEAT & POULTRY

- 1¼ pounds beef flank steak
- 1 pound skinless, boneless chicken-breast halves
- 1 pound pork tenderloin
- 1 pound lean ground turkey
- 2 ounces lean lower-sodium ham
- 3 ounces sliced smoked turkey breast

DAIRY

- 1½ ounces reduced-fat feta cheese
- 3 ounces part-skim mozzarella cheese
- 1 slice reduced-fat Swiss cheese

GRAIN PRODUCTS

- 12 ounces whole-grain fusilli pasta
- 1 package (8.8 ounces) precooked brown rice

CANNED GOODS

- 1 can (15 ounces) black beans
- 1 can (15 ounces) no-salt-added garbanzo beans (chickpeas)

FROZEN

- 2 Van's 8 Whole Grains waffles
- 7 Applegate Farms chicken nuggets
- 1 Healthy Choice Italian Sausage Pasta Bake meal
- 1¼ cups shelled edamame

MISCELLANEOUS

- ⅔ cup hummus
- 2 slices whole-grain melba toast
- 25 SunChips
- 15 sweet potato chips

WEEK 1
BEFORE YOU BEGIN...

We set aside these pages specifically for a one-time writing exercise modeled on results from a 2012 Renison University College study. Researchers from this Canadian school had a group of college-age women spend 15 minutes—just once—writing about the values they believed were most important. The women then went on to lose an average of 3½ pounds in 10 weeks (a control group gained almost 3 pounds on average). "Reflecting on important values can improve self-image, hampering the eat-to-feel-better impulse," says Christine Logel, Ph.D., an author of the study.

So before you get started, take some time to think about things you value. These may include honesty, compassion, a sense of humor—all qualities that can serve you well as you embark upon this seven-week program.

DAY 1

TO-DO LIST

- Read your pledge.

- Assess your schedule for today. Is anything going to make it difficult to stick to your diet? Strategize to overcome obstacles.

- Put some formal exercise on today's calendar or think about ways you can move your body.

- Plan for tomorrow's meals tonight. What are you going to eat? Do you have everything you need? If you're brown-bagging tomorrow's lunch, save time by assembling what you can now.

- Pack your journal or make sure you have a pen and paper (or a smartphone) for making notes throughout the day.

- Remind yourself of the commitment you made—and of how great you're going to feel as you make progress.

STICK-TO-IT STRATEGY

How Do You Define Change? One of the secrets of making a long-lasting transformation is reframing the way you think about it. Instead of seeing change as a process of giving up things you love and doing without, think of it as an exciting means of discovering new things and gaining significant physical, psychological, or emotional advantages. Change is good!

BREAKFAST

Hunger Level*

FOOD/AMOUNT _____

_____
_____
_____
_____

EMOTIONS _____

_____
_____
_____
_____

* See "How to Use This Workbook," p. 13, for guidance on how to score your hunger level.

LUNCH

Hunger Level

FOOD/AMOUNT _____

_____

_____

_____

_____

EMOTIONS _____

_____

_____

_____

_____

========================= TESTER TIP =========================

"How did I get ready to diet? I cleaned out my pantry and fridge, made a vision board with pictures of clothes I wanted to fit into, and broke up with the drive-through clerk at McDonald's!"

—Jeanne Fishwick, 8 pounds and 2¾ inches lost

DINNER

Hunger Level

FOOD/AMOUNT _____

_____

_____

_____

_____

EMOTIONS _____

_____

_____

_____

_____

SNACK 1

Hunger Level

TIME/PLACE _____

FOOD/AMOUNT _____

EMOTIONS _____

SNACK 2

Hunger Level

TIME/PLACE _____

FOOD/AMOUNT _____

EMOTIONS _____

UNPLANNED EATING

Hunger Level

FOOD/AMOUNT _____

TIME/PLACE _____

EMOTIONS _____

DAILY MOVEMENT

Type of Activity	Minutes/Amount	How It Felt
AEROBIC Exercises:		
STRENGTHENING Exercises:		
FLEXIBILITY Exercises:		
BALANCE Exercises:		
INCIDENTAL MOVEMENT		

Meditate Your Way to a Slimmer Body What does meditation have to do with weight loss? A lot, if you're a stress eater. Meditation can help you stay calm in tense and taxing situations. Try this practice from the mindfulness tradition. Begin with 10 minutes a day as your goal and work up to 20.

1. **Sit quietly in a comfortable position.** Close your eyes and relax.

2. **Become aware of your breathing.** Breathe slowly and naturally, drawing air into your belly and exhaling.

3. **Keep focusing on your breathing.** Any time your mind wanders, take note of it and bring your focus back to your breathing. Acknowledge your thoughts, but don't judge them.

4. **When you are finished, sit quietly for a minute,** then open your eyes and rise slowly.

DAILY ASSESSMENT

- This week, the diet is new for you. Did you plan well so that following the day's menu was easy? If you hit any roadblocks, how can you avoid them tomorrow?

- Did you schedule in exercise and stick with it? If not, what changed your plans?

- Did you discover anything about food/movement/yourself today that you found helpful or motivating?

- What nice thing did you do for yourself today?

- Final thoughts on the day: Are you pleased with how the day went? What went well? What do you resolve to change tomorrow?

✻ DON'T FORGET | *Check your to-do list before signing off for the night! It'll help you be ready for tomorrow.*

TO-DO LIST

- Assess your schedule for today. Is anything going to make it difficult to stick to your diet? Strategize to overcome obstacles.

- Put some formal exercise on today's calendar or think about extra ways you can move your body.

- Plan for tomorrow's meals tonight. What are you going to eat? Do you have everything you need? If you're brown-bagging tomorrow's lunch, save time by assembling what you can now.

- Pack your journal or make sure you have a pen and paper (or a smartphone) for making notes throughout the day.

- Remind yourself of the commitment you made—and of how great you're going to feel as you make progress.

MOVE MORE, LOSE MORE

Exercise's Appetite-Control Bonus It's not an accident that avid exercisers tend to be healthy eaters. In a recent review, Harvard researchers proposed that exercise induces changes in the brain that could help people make better food choices. One's power over the drive to eat is controlled by an area of the brain that is constantly bombarded by enticements. But exercise may give that part of your brain a boost, making it easier to say no to tempting treats.

BREAKFAST

Hunger Level

FOOD/AMOUNT _____

EMOTIONS _____

LUNCH

Hunger Level

FOOD/AMOUNT _____

_____

_____

_____

_____

_____

_____

EMOTIONS _____

_____

_____

_____

_____

_____

DINNER

Hunger Level

FOOD/AMOUNT _____

_____

_____

_____

_____

_____

_____

EMOTIONS _____

_____

_____

_____

_____

_____

SNACK 1

Hunger Level

TIME/PLACE _____

FOOD/AMOUNT _____

EMOTIONS _____

SNACK 2

Hunger Level

TIME/PLACE _____

FOOD/AMOUNT _____

EMOTIONS _____

UNPLANNED EATING

Hunger Level

FOOD/AMOUNT _____

TIME/PLACE _____

EMOTIONS _____

DAILY MOVEMENT

Type of Activity	Minutes/Amount	How It Felt
AEROBIC Exercises:		
STRENGTHENING Exercises:		
FLEXIBILITY Exercises:		
BALANCE Exercises:		
INCIDENTAL MOVEMENT		

The Brown-Bag Benefit When you're busy at work or consumed with shuffling kids to and fro, it's easy to forget about lunch. But don't congratulate yourself for missing a meal—it can lead you to go overboard on calories later in the day. The best thing you can do is eat a lunch you packed yourself. There's no harm in going out for lunch occasionally, but there's also no doubt that brown-bagging it contributes to the best weight-loss results. A study at Fred Hutchinson Cancer Research Center in Seattle found that of 123 women dieters followed for a year, those who packed their lunches lost five pounds more than those who dined out for lunch at least once a week.

DAILY ASSESSMENT

● Did you plan well so that following the day's menu was easy? If you hit any roadblocks, how can you avoid them tomorrow?

_____

_____

● Did you schedule in exercise and stick with it? If not, what changed your plans?

_____

_____

● Did you discover anything about food/movement/yourself today that you found helpful or motivating?

_____

_____

● What nice thing did you do for yourself today?

_____

_____

● Final thoughts on the day: Are you pleased with how the day went? What went well? What do you resolve to improve tomorrow?

_____

_____

_____

_____

_____

_____

✻ **DON'T FORGET** | *Check your to-do list before signing off for the night! It'll help you be ready for tomorrow.*

TO-DO LIST

- Assess your schedule for today. Is anything going to make it difficult to stick to your diet? Strategize to overcome obstacles.

- Put some formal exercise on today's calendar or think about extra ways you can move your body.

- Plan for tomorrow's meals tonight. What are you going to eat? Do you have everything you need? If you're brown-bagging tomorrow's lunch, save time by assembling what you can now.

- Pack your journal or make sure you have a pen and paper (or a smartphone) for making notes throughout the day.

- Remind yourself of the commitment you made—and of how great you're going to feel as you make progress.

CRAVINGS CONTROL

Relive the Experience Thinking about what you ate earlier in the day may make you inclined to eat less as the day wears on. So don't just write about your meal—go back and read about it. If you're like participants in a British study, reminiscing about breakfast may help you eat fewer calories at lunch; recalling lunch may help you be satisfied with less at dinner.

BREAKFAST

Hunger Level

FOOD/AMOUNT _____

EMOTIONS _____

LUNCH

Hunger Level

FOOD/AMOUNT _____

_____

_____

_____

_____

_____

_____

EMOTIONS _____

_____

_____

_____

_____

_____

DINNER

Hunger Level

FOOD/AMOUNT _____

_____

_____

_____

_____

_____

_____

EMOTIONS _____

_____

_____

_____

_____

_____

SNACK 1

Hunger Level

TIME/PLACE _____

FOOD/AMOUNT _____

EMOTIONS _____

SNACK 2

Hunger Level

TIME/PLACE _____

FOOD/AMOUNT _____

EMOTIONS _____

UNPLANNED EATING

Hunger Level

FOOD/AMOUNT _____

TIME/PLACE _____

EMOTIONS _____

DAILY MOVEMENT

Type of Activity	Minutes/Amount	How It Felt
AEROBIC Exercises:		
STRENGTHENING Exercises:		
FLEXIBILITY Exercises:		
BALANCE Exercises:		
INCIDENTAL MOVEMENT		

Pile on the Polyphenols By following the 7 *Years Younger Anti-Aging Breakthrough Diet,* you're getting a large daily dose of antioxidants, a potent weapon against aging. One family of antioxidants, the polyphenols, are particularly powerful. Research shows that they inhibit the inflammation and tissue damage associated with aging. One great source of polyphenols: whole grains, especially whole-grain cold cereals and popcorn.

DAILY ASSESSMENT

● Did you plan well so that following the menu plan was easy? If you hit any roadblocks, how can you avoid them tomorrow?

_____

_____

● Did you schedule in exercise and stick with it? If not, what changed your plans?

_____

_____

● Did you discover anything about food/movement/yourself today that you found helpful or motivating?

_____

_____

● What nice thing did you do for yourself today?

_____

_____

● Final thoughts on the day: Are you pleased with how the day went? What went well? What do you resolve to change tomorrow?

_____

_____

_____

_____

_____

_____

_____

_____

✻ **DON'T FORGET** | *Check your to-do list before signing off for the night! It'll help you be ready for tomorrow.*

DAY 4

TO-DO LIST

- Assess your schedule for today. Is anything going to make it difficult to stick to your diet? Strategize to overcome obstacles.

- Put some formal exercise on today's calendar or think about extra ways you can move your body.

- Plan for tomorrow's meals tonight. What are you going to eat? Do you have everything you need? If you're brown-bagging tomorrow's lunch, save time by assembling what you can now.

- Pack your journal or make sure you have a pen and paper (or a smartphone) for making notes throughout the day.

- Remind yourself of the commitment you made—and of how great you're going to feel as you make progress.

MOVE MORE, LOSE MORE

Cool It Keeping cool while you exercise can help you stick to your routine, increase your pace, and burn more calories. That's what a Stanford University study found, using a cooling device: The women in the study dropped an average of three inches from their waists and lowered their blood pressures over a period of 12 weeks. You can duplicate the effect by sipping ice-cold water as you work out.

BREAKFAST

Hunger Level

FOOD/AMOUNT _____

_____

_____

_____

_____

_____

EMOTIONS _____

_____

_____

_____

_____

LUNCH

FOOD/AMOUNT _____

_____

_____

_____

_____

_____

_____

EMOTIONS _____

_____

_____

_____

_____

_____

DINNER

Hunger
Level

FOOD/AMOUNT _____

_____

_____

_____

_____

_____

_____

EMOTIONS _____

_____

_____

_____

_____

_____

SNACK 1

Hunger Level

TIME/PLACE _____

FOOD/AMOUNT _____

EMOTIONS _____

SNACK 2

Hunger Level

TIME/PLACE _____

FOOD/AMOUNT _____

EMOTIONS _____

UNPLANNED EATING

Hunger Level

FOOD/AMOUNT _____

TIME/PLACE _____

EMOTIONS _____

DAILY MOVEMENT

Type of Activity	Minutes/Amount	How It Felt
AEROBIC Exercises:		
STRENGTHENING Exercises:		
FLEXIBILITY Exercises:		
BALANCE Exercises:		
INCIDENTAL MOVEMENT		

Should You Weigh Yourself? GHRI Nutrition Director Samantha Cassetty, M.S., R.D., responds with an unequivocal "yes." Stepping on the scale daily, or at least two or three times a week, helps you discover what's working and what's not. Bear in mind that your weight may fluctuate a little, but if the numbers on the scale aren't budging or are inching back up after you've already lost weight, it's a sign that you need to scrutinize your eating more closely. Once you've completed the seven-week diet, continue to weigh yourself. If you gain as much as five pounds, hop back on the plan again.

DAILY ASSESSMENT

- Did you plan well so that following the menu plan was easy? If you hit any roadblocks, how can you avoid them tomorrow?

_____

_____

- Did you schedule in exercise and stick with it? If not, what changed your plans?

_____

_____

- Did you discover anything about food/movement/yourself today that you found helpful or motivating?

_____

_____

- What nice thing did you do for yourself today?

_____

_____

- Final thoughts on the day: Are you pleased with how the day went? What went well? What do you resolve to change tomorrow?

_____

_____

_____

_____

_____

_____

| ✳ **DON'T FORGET** | _Check your to-do list before signing off for the night! It'll help you be ready for tomorrow._ |

TO-DO LIST

- Assess your schedule for today. Is anything going to make it difficult to stick to your diet? Strategize to overcome obstacles.

- Put some formal exercise on today's calendar or think about extra ways you can move your body.

- Plan for tomorrow's meals tonight. What are you going to eat? Do you have everything you need? If you're brown-bagging tomorrow's lunch, save time by assembling what you can now.

- Pack your journal or make sure you have a pen and paper (or a smartphone) for making notes throughout the day.

- Remind yourself of the commitment you made—and of how great you're going to feel as you make progress.

MORE MINDFUL EATING

In Search of Saboteurs Every time you eat when you're not hungry just to satisfy someone else—or feel you have an excuse for eating extra because you're only being considerate—you're sabotaging your health. As you write in this workbook, explore the saboteur conundrum. Learning to say no will be a lot easier if you can pinpoint episodes in which "yes" led you down the wrong path.

BREAKFAST

Hunger Level

FOOD/AMOUNT _____

_____

_____

_____

_____

EMOTIONS _____

_____

_____

_____

_____

LUNCH

Hunger Level

FOOD/AMOUNT _____

_____
_____
_____
_____

EMOTIONS _____

_____
_____
_____
_____

DINNER

Hunger Level

FOOD/AMOUNT _____

_____
_____
_____
_____
_____

EMOTIONS _____

_____
_____
_____

SNACK 1

Hunger Level

TIME/PLACE _____

FOOD/AMOUNT _____

EMOTIONS _____

SNACK 2

Hunger Level

TIME/PLACE _____

FOOD/AMOUNT _____

EMOTIONS _____

UNPLANNED EATING

Hunger Level

FOOD/AMOUNT _____

TIME/PLACE _____

EMOTIONS _____

DAILY MOVEMENT

Type of Activity	Minutes/Amount	How It Felt
AEROBIC Exercises:		
STRENGTHENING Exercises:		
FLEXIBILITY Exercises:		
BALANCE Exercises:		
INCIDENTAL MOVEMENT		

Salad Swaps Greens are great—unless you load up a salad with a lot of fattening extras. Here are some lower-calorie alternatives.

INSTEAD OF...	CHOOSE	CALORIES SAVED
¹/₂ cup croutons (61 cals.)	3 pita chips (39 cals.)	22
¹/₄ cup Cheddar cheese (114 cals.)	¹/₄ cup low-fat mozzarella (85 cals.)	29
¹/₂ cup tuna salad (192 cals.)	¹/₂ cup tuna fish, chunked (66 cals.)	126
2 Tbsp. ranch dressing (145 cals.)	2 Tbsp. salsa (10 cals.)	135

DAILY ASSESSMENT

● Did you plan well so that following the day's menu was easy? If you hit any roadblocks, how can you avoid them tomorrow?

● Did you schedule in exercise and stick with it? If not, what changed your plans?

● Did you discover anything about food/movement/yourself today that you found helpful or motivating?

● What nice thing did you do for yourself today?

● Final thoughts on the day: Are you pleased with how the day went? What went well? What do you resolve to change tomorrow?

✱ **DON'T FORGET** | *Check your to-do list before signing off for the night! It'll help you be ready for tomorrow.*

TO-DO LIST

- Assess your schedule for today. Is anything going to make it difficult to stick to your diet? Strategize to overcome obstacles.

- Put some formal exercise on today's calendar or think about extra ways you can move your body.

- Plan for tomorrow's meals tonight. What are you going to eat? Do you have everything you need? If you're brown-bagging tomorrow's lunch, save time by assembling what you can now.

- Pack your journal or make sure you have a pen and paper (or a smartphone) for making notes throughout the day.

- Remind yourself of the commitment you made—and of how great you're going to feel as you make progress.

ANTI-AGING EATING

Bean There If you eat just half a cup of beans a day, you can potentially slash your "bad" LDL cholesterol 8% or more in eight weeks—and every 1% drop in LDL can lower heart disease risk by up to 3%. Beans are rich in saponins—phytochemicals that, at least in the lab, inhibit cancer-cell reproduction. That means they may help prevent cancer in the body, too.

BREAKFAST

Hunger Level

FOOD/AMOUNT _____

_____
_____
_____
_____
_____

EMOTIONS _____

_____
_____
_____
_____

LUNCH

Hunger Level

FOOD/AMOUNT _____

_____

_____

_____

_____

_____

EMOTIONS _____

_____

_____

_____

_____

_____

DINNER

Hunger Level

FOOD/AMOUNT _____

_____

_____

_____

_____

_____

EMOTIONS _____

_____

_____

_____

_____

_____

SNACK 1

TIME/PLACE _____ *Hunger Level*

FOOD/AMOUNT _____

EMOTIONS _____

SNACK 2

TIME/PLACE _____ *Hunger Level*

FOOD/AMOUNT _____

EMOTIONS _____

UNPLANNED EATING

FOOD/AMOUNT _____ *Hunger Level*

TIME/PLACE _____

EMOTIONS _____

DAILY MOVEMENT

Type of Activity	Minutes/Amount	How It Felt
AEROBIC Exercises:		
STRENGTHENING Exercises:		
FLEXIBILITY Exercises:		
BALANCE Exercises:		
INCIDENTAL MOVEMENT		

Go the Extra Mile (or Even Just a Few Steps)

- Get up and talk to colleagues down the hall instead of sending e-mails.
- Walk, don't drive, to the mailbox to send off letters and bill payments.
- Get your kids to hoof it to school—it will benefit all of you.
- Pace the room while talking on the phone.
- Take a walk around the block after each time you eat, even if you've only had a snack.

DAILY ASSESSMENT

- Did you plan well so that following the day's menu was easy? If you hit any roadblocks, how can you avoid them tomorrow?

_____

_____

- Did you schedule in exercise and stick with it? If not, what changed your plans?

_____

_____

- Did you discover anything about food/movement/yourself today that you found helpful or motivating?

_____

_____

- What nice thing did you do for yourself today?

_____

_____

- Final thoughts on the day: Are you pleased with how the day went? What went well? What do you resolve to change tomorrow?

_____

_____

✳ **DON'T FORGET** | *Check your to-do list before signing off for the night! It'll help you be ready for tomorrow.*

TO-DO LIST

- Assess your schedule for today. Is anything going to make it difficult to stick to your diet? Strategize to overcome obstacles.

- Put some formal exercise on today's calendar or think about extra ways you can move your body.

- Plan for tomorrow's meals tonight. What are you going to eat? Do you have everything you need? If you're brown-bagging tomorrow's lunch, save time by assembling what you can now.

- Pack your journal or make sure you have a pen and paper (or a smartphone) for making notes throughout the day.

- Remind yourself of the commitment you made–and of how great you're going to feel as you make progress.

CRAVINGS CONTROL

Getting Back on the Wagon When a day, or even a week, goes badly and you find yourself off the diet track, try what behavior specialist M.J. Ryan calls the Four A's: **1.** Assess the current situation. **2.** Adjust what needs to be done. **3.** Admire yourself for being strong enough to start again. **4.** Act quickly to implement your new course of action.

BREAKFAST

Hunger Level

FOOD/AMOUNT _____

_____
_____
_____
_____
_____

EMOTIONS _____

_____
_____
_____

LUNCH

Hunger Level

FOOD/AMOUNT _____

_____

_____

_____

_____

_____

_____

EMOTIONS _____

_____

_____

_____

_____

_____

DINNER

Hunger Level

FOOD/AMOUNT _____

_____

_____

_____

_____

_____

_____

EMOTIONS _____

_____

_____

_____

_____

_____

SNACK 1

Hunger Level

TIME/PLACE _____

FOOD/AMOUNT _____

EMOTIONS _____

SNACK 2

Hunger Level

TIME/PLACE _____

FOOD/AMOUNT _____

EMOTIONS _____

UNPLANNED EATING

Hunger Level

FOOD/AMOUNT _____

TIME/PLACE _____

EMOTIONS _____

DAILY MOVEMENT

Type of Activity	Minutes/Amount	How It Felt
AEROBIC Exercises:		
STRENGTHENING Exercises:		
FLEXIBILITY Exercises:		
BALANCE Exercises:		
INCIDENTAL MOVEMENT		

Build a Better Sandwich Choose whole-grain bread (not a big roll), load up on veggies, and limit meat to 100 calories, cheese to 50 calories, and spread to 50 calories or less. Here's how some spreads line up.

SPREAD	CALORIES PER TABLESPOON
Light mayonnaise	45
Honey mustard	30
Hummus	23
Ketchup	15
Mustard	9

DAILY ASSESSMENT

● Did you plan well so that following the day's menu was easy? If you hit any roadblocks, how can you avoid them tomorrow?

● Did you schedule in exercise and stick with it? If not, what changed your plans?

● Did you discover anything about food/movement/yourself today that you found helpful or motivating?

● What nice thing did you do for yourself today?

● Final thoughts on the day: Are you pleased with how the day went? What went well? What do you resolve to change tomorrow?

❋ **DON'T FORGET** | *Check your to-do list before signing off for the night! It'll help you be ready for tomorrow.*

How Was Your Week?

The beginning of a diet can seem relatively easy: You're excited and highly motivated, so the first week has the potential to go very well. Was that true for you? If so, what can you do to keep yourself pumped up? If things didn't go as well as you expected, write about what was particularly challenging and what you might do to work on the obstacles you encountered.

_____

_____

_____

_____

_____

_____

_____

_____

_____

_____

GOALS FOR NEXT WEEK

_____

_____

_____

_____

_____

_____

_____

_____

_____

_____

WEEK 2

This week and in the remaining weeks, you'll be working snacks (larger ones for men) into your day. That bumps calories up to a satisfying 1,450 for women, 1,575 for slightly to moderately active men, and 1,700 for highly active men.

WEEK 2

MEAL PLAN

DAY 1
Breakfast: New York Bagel
Lunch: Mediterranean Vegetarian Wrap
Snack 1: Movie Mix
Dinner: Steak Sandwich with
Grilled Onions
Snack 2: Cheese Bite

DAY 2
Breakfast: Ham & Veggie Hash
Lunch: Protein Plate
Snack 1: Iced-Coffee Break
Dinner: Shrimp & Fresh Corn Grits
Snack 2: Honeydew "Sundae"

DAY 3
Breakfast: Peach Melba Yogurt
Lunch: Roast Beef Pockets
Snack 1: Pistachios
Dinner: Chicken Lo Mein Primavera
Snack 2: Cherries & Cheese

DAY 4
Breakfast: Breakfast Pizza
Lunch: Spicy Black Bean Soup
Snack 1: Strawberry Sipper
Dinner: Almond-Crusted Tilapia
Snack 2: Out & About

DAY 5
Breakfast: 5-Minute Multigrain Cereal
Lunch: Shrimp Caesar Salad
Snack 1: Pineapple Plate
Dinner: Spice-Rubbed
Pork Tenderloin
Snack 2: Prosciutto & Mozzarella Plate

DAY 6
Breakfast: Berry Blast Breakfast Shake
Lunch: Grilled Chicken Sandwich
Snack 1: Chips & Cheese
Dinner: Spaghetti with Pesto Verde
Snack 2: Pudding Parfait

DAY 7
Breakfast: Huevos Rancheros
Lunch: Sushi to Go
Snack 1: Veggies & Dill Dip
Dinner: Healthy-Makeover Meatloaf
Snack 2: Blueberry Lassi

Shopping List

For breakfasts, lunches, and dinners serving anywhere from one to six. Check recipes to make adjustments depending on the number of people you are feeding.

FRESH PRODUCE

- 1 bunch basil
- 1 tablespoon chives
- ¾ cup cilantro leaves
- 1 teaspoon dill
- 1 tablespoon mint leaves
- ¼ cup flat-leaf parsley leaves
- 1 teaspoon thyme leaves
- 18 grape or cherry tomatoes
- 6 regular tomatoes
- 2 bags (5 to 6 ounces each) mixed salad greens or baby arugula
- 1 head romaine lettuce
- 6 ounces baby spinach
- 6 baby carrots
- 2 large carrots
- 4 stalks celery
- 5 cups fresh corn kernels (from about 8 ears)
- 2½ pounds green beans
- 1 package (10 ounces) sliced white mushrooms
- 1 medium and 2 large red bell peppers
- 6 medium red potatoes (1½ pounds total)
- 1 small yellow summer squash
- 15 sugar snap peas
- 3 medium and 1 large zucchini
- 2 avocados
- 1 small apple
- 1 banana
- 1 pint (12 ounces) blackberries
- ¼ cup cantaloupe chunks
- 20 cherries
- 5 grapes
- 1 honeydew melon
- 1 small orange
- 2 peaches
- 2 pears
- ½ cup pineapple chunks
- 2 teaspoons pomegranate seeds
- ⅓ cup raspberries
- 1 pint (12 ounces) strawberries

SEAFOOD

- 12 ounces (20- to 23-count) large raw shrimp, shelled and deveined
- 4 tilapia fillets (1½ pounds total)
- 1 ounce lox
- 8 large precooked shrimp
- 1 (6-piece) California maki sushi roll (made with brown rice, if available)*

MEAT & POULTRY

- 1¼ pounds beef flank steak
- 1 pound pork tenderloin
- 2 pounds lean ground turkey
- 2 ounces lean roast beef
- 1 ounce low-sodium smoked turkey breast
- 4 ounces thick-sliced ham or 4-ounce piece of ham
- ½ ounce very thinly sliced prosciutto
- 1 link (3 ounces) fully cooked andouille sausage

DAIRY

- 1 Mini Babybel Sharp Original or Gouda cheese
- 2 slices reduced-fat Cheddar cheese
- 1 ounce reduced-fat feta cheese
- ¾ ounce aged goat cheese or Brie
- 2 ounces part-skim mozzarella cheese
- 2 sticks part-skim mozzarella string cheese

Buy the day you'll be eating it.

½ cup low-fat (1%), low-sodium
cottage cheese

1 container (6 ounces) sugar-free
vanilla pudding

1 container (6 ounces) low-fat or
nonfat plain yogurt

GRAIN PRODUCTS

1 package (9 ounces) fresh whole-
grain linguine

¼ cup whole wheat orzo pasta

8 ounces whole-grain spaghetti

1 loaf whole-grain sourdough bread

½ cup quick-cooking grits

1 package (8.8 ounces) Uncle Ben's
Ready Rice brown rice

CANNED GOODS

3 cans (15 ounces each) black beans

1 can (14½ ounces) chicken broth

1 can (28 ounces) whole peeled
tomatoes in juice

FROZEN FOODS

2 cups frozen sliced blueberries,
strawberries, or berry medley

1 package (10 ounces) frozen
broccoli florets

MISCELLANEOUS

1 Kind Mini Fruit & Nut Delight Bar

½ cup hummus

½ cup Edy's/Dreyer's Slow Churned
No Sugar Added Ice Cream,
vanilla flavor

1 cup Imagine Creamy Portobello
Mushroom Soup

1 cup Good Health Half Naked
Popcorn

6 sweet potato chips

1 package (14 ounces) extra-firm tofu

1 can (11½ ounces) low-sodium
tomato or vegetable juice

5 Food Should Taste Good
Multigrain tortilla chips

3 reduced-fat Triscuits

DAY 1

TO-DO LIST

- Reread your pledge.

- Assess your schedule for today. Is anything going to make it difficult to stick to your diet? Strategize to overcome obstacles.

- Put some formal exercise on today's calendar or think about ways you can move your body.

- Plan for tomorrow's meals tonight. What are you going to eat? Do you have everything you need? If you're brown-bagging tomorrow's lunch, save time by assembling what you can now.

- Pack your journal or make sure you have a pen and paper (or a smartphone) for making notes throughout the day.

- Remind yourself of the commitment you made—and of how great you're going to feel as you make progress.

STICK-TO-IT STRATEGY

Set Your Schedule Following this program requires time—make sure you have it mapped out in your schedule. Think of exercise and cooking and shopping for your meals as you would any other commitments, and note them on your calendar. Also be certain that the people in your life are on board, so they give you the time and space you need to accomplish your goals.

BREAKFAST

Hunger Level

FOOD/AMOUNT _____

_____

_____

_____

_____

EMOTIONS _____

_____

_____

_____

_____

_____

LUNCH

Hunger
Level

FOOD/AMOUNT _____

_____

_____

_____

_____

EMOTIONS _____

_____

_____

_____

_____

=========== TESTER TIP ===========

"If you tell yourself you can do anything, if you believe
in yourself and say to yourself internally, *I can do this,
I will succeed, I am doing this, I can do anything
that anyone else has done before me,* you will succeed."

—*Maria Arap, 10½ pounds and 2¼ inches lost*

DINNER

Hunger
Level

FOOD/AMOUNT _____

_____

_____

_____

_____

EMOTIONS _____

_____

_____

_____

_____

SNACK 1

Hunger Level

TIME/PLACE _____

FOOD/AMOUNT _____

EMOTIONS _____

SNACK 2

Hunger Level

TIME/PLACE _____

FOOD/AMOUNT _____

EMOTIONS _____

UNPLANNED EATING

Hunger Level

FOOD/AMOUNT _____

TIME/PLACE _____

EMOTIONS _____

DAILY MOVEMENT

Type of Activity	Minutes/Amount	How It Felt
AEROBIC Exercises:		
STRENGTHENING Exercises:		
FLEXIBILITY Exercises:		
BALANCE Exercises:		
INCIDENTAL MOVEMENT		

Emotional-Eater Alert

Stress-Snacking Prevention You're stressed, you're emotional—but are you really hungry? When you find yourself at that moment of truth—will you have that bowl of ice cream or won't you?—pause. Ask yourself if you're really hungry and, if not, have an emotionally nurturing alternative at the ready. To prepare for these critical times, write down:

- **The name of a family member or friend you can call and vent to instead of eating:**

  _____

- **A binge-prevention meditation or breathing technique to try:**

  _____

- **An activity to busy your hands with (e.g., knitting, puzzles):**

  _____

DAILY ASSESSMENT

- Compare how well you did on the diet today with how well you did last week. Has anything changed? Are you finding certain things hard to stick with? If so, think about why and work on ways to either remove roadblocks or improve your willpower.

  _____

- Did you schedule in exercise and follow through? If not, what changed your plans?

  _____

- Did you discover anything about food/movement/yourself today that you found helpful or motivating?

  _____

- What nice thing did you do for yourself today?

  _____

- Final thoughts on the day: Are you pleased with how the day went? What went well? What do you resolve to change tomorrow?

  _____

  _____

  _____

✱ DON'T FORGET | *Check your to-do list before signing off for the night! It'll help you be ready for tomorrow.*

DAY 2

TO-DO LIST

- Assess your schedule for today. Is anything going to make it difficult to stick to your diet? Strategize to overcome obstacles.

- Put some formal exercise on today's calendar or think about extra ways you can move your body.

- Plan for tomorrow's meals tonight. What are you going to eat? Do you have everything you need? If you're brown-bagging tomorrow's lunch, save time by assembling what you can now.

- Pack your journal or make sure you have a pen and paper (or a smartphone) for making notes throughout the day.

- Remind yourself of the commitment you made—and of how great you're going to feel as you make progress.

MINDLESS-MUNCHER ALERT

Party Policy It's difficult to unthinkingly eat hors d'oeuvres when your hands are full. At parties, carry a clutch purse in one hand and hold a glass of sparkling water in the other. You might even designate yourself the gathering's photographer so you can have an excuse to carry your smartphone or camera in one hand.

BREAKFAST

Hunger Level

FOOD/AMOUNT _____

_____

_____

_____

_____

EMOTIONS _____

_____

_____

_____

LUNCH

Hunger
Level

FOOD/AMOUNT _____

_____
_____
_____
_____
_____
_____
_____

EMOTIONS _____

_____
_____
_____
_____
_____

DINNER

Hunger
Level

FOOD/AMOUNT _____

_____
_____
_____
_____
_____
_____

EMOTIONS _____

_____
_____
_____
_____
_____

SNACK 1

Hunger Level

TIME/PLACE _____

FOOD/AMOUNT _____

EMOTIONS _____

SNACK 2

Hunger Level

TIME/PLACE _____

FOOD/AMOUNT _____

EMOTIONS _____

UNPLANNED EATING

Hunger Level

FOOD/AMOUNT _____

TIME/PLACE _____

EMOTIONS _____

DAILY MOVEMENT

Type of Activity	Minutes/Amount	How It Felt
AEROBIC Exercises:		
STRENGTHENING Exercises:		
FLEXIBILITY Exercises:		
BALANCE Exercises:		
INCIDENTAL MOVEMENT		

Move More, Lose More

Boredom Buster Here's a way to get fit and avoid the tedium of doing the same workout every day. Fill a "Fit Game Jar" with instructions for 15 to 20 different workouts you have created or found on various fitness websites and in magazines (include the workouts from the 7 *Years Younger Anti-Aging Breakthrough Diet*, of course). "They can range from swim workouts to group exercise classes to the latest exercise trend," says Erin Kreitz Shirey, CEO/master trainer of Power Fitness PDX and creator of the blog *Dig Deep, Play Hard*, who came up with the Fit Game Jar idea. Every day (or every other day), select a different workout from the jar to do that day. The jar should be empty by month's end.

DAILY ASSESSMENT

● Run an attitude check on yourself: Were you having any negative ("I'm angry at myself for eating that") or defeatist ("I don't have any willpower; I should just give up") thoughts today?

_____

_____

● Did you schedule in exercise and stick with it? If not, what changed your plans?

_____

_____

● Did you discover anything about food/movement/yourself today that you found helpful or motivating?

_____

_____

● What nice thing did you do for yourself today?

_____

_____

● Final thoughts on the day: Are you pleased with how the day went? What went well? What do you resolve to improve tomorrow?

_____

_____

_____

_____

_____

| **✱ DON'T FORGET** | *Check your to-do list before signing off for the night! It'll help you be ready for tomorrow.* |

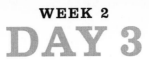

TO-DO LIST

- Assess your schedule for today. Is anything going to make it difficult to stick to your diet? Strategize to overcome obstacles.

- Put some formal exercise on today's calendar or think about extra ways you can move your body.

- Plan for tomorrow's meals tonight. What are you going to eat? Do you have everything you need? If you're brown-bagging tomorrow's lunch, save time by assembling what you can now.

- Pack your journal or make sure you have a pen and paper (or a smartphone) for making notes throughout the day.

- Remind yourself of the commitment you made—and of how great you're going to feel as you make progress.

ANTI-AGING EATING

Live-Longer Foods Compare apples and oranges, and you'll find that they both are good sources of rutin, an antioxidant that researchers at Harvard Medical School found has anticlotting properties. Preventing clots helps prevent heart attack and stroke. Beyond raiding the fruit bowl, you can get more rutin in your diet by drinking tea and eating berries.

BREAKFAST

Hunger Level

FOOD/AMOUNT _____

_____
_____
_____
_____
_____

EMOTIONS _____

_____
_____
_____
_____

LUNCH

Hunger Level

FOOD/AMOUNT _____

_____

_____

_____

_____

_____

_____

_____

EMOTIONS _____

_____

_____

_____

_____

_____

DINNER

Hunger Level

FOOD/AMOUNT _____

_____

_____

_____

_____

_____

_____

_____

EMOTIONS _____

_____

_____

_____

_____

_____

SNACK 1

Hunger Level

TIME/PLACE _____

FOOD/AMOUNT _____

EMOTIONS _____

SNACK 2

Hunger Level

TIME/PLACE _____

FOOD/AMOUNT _____

EMOTIONS _____

UNPLANNED EATING

Hunger Level

FOOD/AMOUNT _____

TIME/PLACE _____

EMOTIONS _____

DAILY MOVEMENT

Type of Activity	Minutes/Amount	How It Felt
AEROBIC Exercises:		
STRENGTHENING Exercises:		
FLEXIBILITY Exercises:		
BALANCE Exercises:		
INCIDENTAL MOVEMENT		

Cravings Control

Surprising Fast-Food Selections Find yourself in a fast-food or chain restaurant? Don't panic. You may be able to do better than you think if you make a good choice—but the best one might not be obvious. In fact, while chicken dishes often seem like the most diet-friendly options, most chains have lower-calorie selections elsewhere on the menu. Here are three cases in point:

CHAIN	CHICKEN OPTION	LIGHTER CHOICE	YOU SAVE...
Panda Express	SweetFire Chicken Breast *(440 cals.)*	Shanghai Angus Steak *(240 cals.)*	**200** calories
Au Bon Pain	Chicken Cobb Salad *(660 cals.)*	Tuna Garden Salad *(400 cals.)*	**260** calories
Outback Steakhouse	Alice Springs Chicken *(1,139 cals.)*	Perfectly Grilled Salmon *(483 cals.)*	**656** calories

DAILY ASSESSMENT

● Run an attitude check on yourself: Were you having any negative ("I'm angry at myself for eating that") or defeatist ("I don't have any willpower; I should just give up") thoughts today?

● Did you schedule in exercise and stick with it? If not, what changed your plans?

● Did you discover anything about food/movement/yourself today that you found helpful or motivating?

● What nice thing did you do for yourself today?

● Final thoughts on the day: Are you pleased with how the day went? What went well? What do you resolve to improve tomorrow?

---

* DON'T FORGET	*Check your to-do list before signing off for the night! It'll help you be ready for tomorrow.*

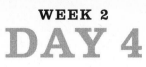

DAY 4

TO-DO LIST

- Assess your schedule for today. Is anything going to make it difficult to stick to your diet? Strategize to overcome obstacles.

- Put some formal exercise on today's calendar or think about extra ways you can move your body.

- Plan for tomorrow's meals tonight. What are you going to eat? Do you have everything you need? If you're brown-bagging tomorrow's lunch, save time by assembling what you can now.

- Pack your journal or make sure you have a pen and paper (or a smartphone) for making notes throughout the day.

- Remind yourself of the commitment you made—and of how great you're going to feel as you make progress.

STICK-TO-IT STRATEGY

Focus on the Journey Even as you daydream about slipping into your skinny jeans, don't lose sight of the day-to-day steps that will get you there. One study found that in a group of 126 overweight women trying to shed pounds, those who concentrated most on daily to-do's were more likely to succeed than those whose attention was on their slimmer future selves. Concentrate on the "how" so you can get to "wow."

BREAKFAST

Hunger Level

FOOD/AMOUNT _____

_____

_____

_____

_____

_____

EMOTIONS _____

_____

_____

_____

_____

LUNCH

*Hunger
Level*

FOOD/AMOUNT _____

_____

_____

_____

_____

_____

_____

EMOTIONS _____

_____

_____

_____

_____

_____

DINNER

*Hunger
Level*

FOOD/AMOUNT _____

_____

_____

_____

_____

_____

_____

EMOTIONS _____

_____

_____

_____

_____

_____

SNACK 1

Hunger Level

TIME/PLACE _____

FOOD/AMOUNT _____

EMOTIONS _____

SNACK 2

Hunger Level

TIME/PLACE _____

FOOD/AMOUNT _____

EMOTIONS _____

UNPLANNED EATING

Hunger Level

FOOD/AMOUNT _____

TIME/PLACE _____

EMOTIONS _____

DAILY MOVEMENT

Type of Activity	Minutes/Amount	How It Felt
AEROBIC Exercises:		
STRENGTHENING Exercises:		
FLEXIBILITY Exercises:		
BALANCE Exercises:		
INCIDENTAL MOVEMENT		

Move More, Lose More

Go Green Maybe what's missing from your workout life is some greenery. In a 2012 study at the Centre for Sports & Exercise Science at the University of Essex in the U.K., cyclists who viewed scenes of green trees in a nature video felt happier and perceived their workouts to be less difficult than cyclists who viewed scenes in black and white or in red. If exercise feels like drudgery, maybe it's time to ditch the treadmill and get outdoors.

DAILY ASSESSMENT

- Run an attitude check on yourself: Were you having any negative ("I'm angry at myself for eating that") or defeatist ("I don't have any willpower; I should just give up") thoughts today?

_____

_____

- Did you schedule in exercise and stick with it? If not, what changed your plans?

_____

_____

- Did you discover anything about food/movement/yourself today that you found helpful or motivating?

_____

_____

- What nice thing did you do for yourself today?

_____

_____

- Final thoughts on the day: Are you pleased with how the day went? What went well? What do you resolve to improve tomorrow?

_____

_____

_____

_____

_____

_____

| ✴ **DON'T FORGET** | _Check your to-do list before signing off for the night! It'll help you be ready for tomorrow._ |

TO-DO LIST

- Assess your schedule for today. Is anything going to make it difficult to stick to your diet? Strategize to overcome obstacles.

- Put some formal exercise on today's calendar or think about extra ways you can move your body.

- Plan for tomorrow's meals tonight. What are you going to eat? Do you have everything you need? If you're brown-bagging tomorrow's lunch, save time by assembling what you can now.

- Pack your journal or make sure you have a pen and paper (or a smartphone) for making notes throughout the day.

- Remind yourself of the commitment you made—and of how great you're going to feel as you make progress.

MORE MINDFUL EATING

The Skinny Way to Eat Here are a few reminders that can really make a difference: Eat slowly, pause between bites, and enjoy the flavor. Notice the texture, the temperature, and the aroma. Is it sweet or savory? Is there spice? Crunchiness? When you eat slowly, eating takes longer, which gives your brain the 20 minutes it needs to signal your stomach when you've had enough.

BREAKFAST

Hunger Level

FOOD/AMOUNT _____

_____
_____
_____
_____

EMOTIONS _____

_____
_____
_____
_____
_____

LUNCH

Hunger Level

FOOD/AMOUNT _____

_____

_____

_____

_____

EMOTIONS _____

_____

_____

_____

_____

=== TESTER TIP ===

"I hung my old jeans on my closet door to inspire me to fit back into them."

—Winston Leung, 24 pounds and 4¾ inches lost

DINNER

Hunger Level

FOOD/AMOUNT _____

_____

_____

_____

_____

_____

_____

EMOTIONS _____

_____

_____

_____

SNACK 1

Hunger Level

TIME/PLACE _____

FOOD/AMOUNT _____

EMOTIONS _____

SNACK 2

Hunger Level

TIME/PLACE _____

FOOD/AMOUNT _____

EMOTIONS _____

UNPLANNED EATING

Hunger Level

FOOD/AMOUNT _____

TIME/PLACE _____

EMOTIONS _____

DAILY MOVEMENT

Type of Activity	Minutes/Amount	How It Felt
AEROBIC Exercises:		
STRENGTHENING Exercises:		
FLEXIBILITY Exercises:		
BALANCE Exercises:		
INCIDENTAL MOVEMENT		

Weight-Loss Booster

50-Calorie Sweet Snacks You can swap one of these snacks for a 50-calorie piece of fruit on occasion.

- Jell-O Sugar-Free Pudding cup
- 5 Dole Nutrition Plus Chia & Fruit Clusters
- 14 frozen grapes
- 1/3 cup raspberries drizzled with 1 teaspoon melted chocolate chips

DAILY ASSESSMENT

- Run an attitude check on yourself: Were you having any negative ("I'm angry at myself for eating that") or defeatist ("I don't have any willpower; I should just give up") thoughts today?

_____

_____

- Did you schedule in exercise and stick with it? If not, what changed your plans?

_____

_____

- Did you discover anything about food/movement/yourself today that you found helpful or motivating?

_____

_____

- What nice thing did you do for yourself today?

_____

_____

- Final thoughts on the day: Are you pleased with how the day went? What went well? What do you resolve to improve tomorrow?

_____

_____

_____

_____

_____

✱ DON'T FORGET | _Check your to-do list before signing off for the night! It'll help you be ready for tomorrow._

TO-DO LIST

- Assess your schedule for today. Is anything going to make it difficult to stick to your diet? Strategize to overcome obstacles.

- Put some formal exercise on today's calendar or think about extra ways you can move your body.

- Plan for tomorrow's meals tonight. What are you going to eat? Do you have everything you need? If you're brown-bagging tomorrow's lunch, save time by assembling what you can now.

- Pack your journal or make sure you have a pen and paper (or a smartphone) for making notes throughout the day.

- Remind yourself of the commitment you made—and of how great you're going to feel as you make progress.

MOVE MORE, LOSE MORE

Fitness Fights Colds When you're down and out with a bad cold, you don't have to feel guilty about missing exercise—you should take it easy. But as your sniffles abate, start moving. Exercise may help clear any lingering congestion and prevent future illness: People who work out regularly get fewer colds. Start slowly—with yoga or walking—if you're not feeling 100% yet.

BREAKFAST

Hunger Level

FOOD/AMOUNT _____

_____

_____

_____

_____

_____

EMOTIONS _____

_____

_____

_____

_____

LUNCH

○ *Hunger Level*

FOOD/AMOUNT _____

_____
_____
_____
_____
_____
_____
_____

EMOTIONS _____

_____
_____
_____
_____
_____

DINNER

○ *Hunger Level*

FOOD/AMOUNT _____

_____
_____
_____
_____
_____
_____
_____

EMOTIONS _____

_____
_____
_____
_____
_____

SNACK 1

TIME/PLACE _____ *Hunger Level*

FOOD/AMOUNT _____

_____

_____

EMOTIONS _____

_____

SNACK 2

TIME/PLACE _____ *Hunger Level*

FOOD/AMOUNT _____

_____

_____

EMOTIONS _____

_____

UNPLANNED EATING

FOOD/AMOUNT _____ *Hunger Level*

_____

_____

_____

_____

TIME/PLACE _____

_____

_____

EMOTIONS _____

_____

_____

_____

_____

_____

_____

_____

_____

_____

DAILY MOVEMENT

Type of Activity	Minutes/Amount	How It Felt
AEROBIC Exercises:		
STRENGTHENING Exercises:		
FLEXIBILITY Exercises:		
BALANCE Exercises:		
INCIDENTAL MOVEMENT		

Anti-Aging Eating

C Is for Complexion Pepper your diet with a top anti-wrinkle food: red, yellow, and orange bell peppers. These bright picks from the garden are bursting with vitamin C, an antioxidant that quenches the free radicals that interfere with collagen production (collagen gives the skin its structure, keeping it "plumped" and wrinkle-free). All the peppers are C-rich, but there are differences: Red peppers have more of it than yellow ones do, and yellow peppers have more than orange ones.

DAILY ASSESSMENT

- Run an attitude check on yourself: Were you having any negative ("I'm angry at myself for eating that") or defeatist ("I don't have any willpower; I should just give up") thoughts today?

- Did you schedule in exercise and stick with it? If not, what changed your plans?

- Did you discover anything about food/movement/yourself today that you found helpful or motivating?

- What nice thing did you do for yourself today?

- Final thoughts on the day: Are you pleased with how the day went? What went well? What do you resolve to improve tomorrow?

❋ DON'T FORGET | *Check your to-do list before signing off for the night! It'll help you be ready for tomorrow.*

DAY 7

TO-DO LIST

- Assess your schedule for today. Is anything going to make it difficult to stick to your diet? Strategize to overcome obstacles.

- Put some formal exercise on today's calendar or think about extra ways you can move your body.

- Plan for tomorrow's meals tonight. What are you going to eat? Do you have everything you need? If you're brown-bagging tomorrow's lunch, save time by assembling what you can now.

- Pack your journal or make sure you have a pen and paper (or a smartphone) for making notes throughout the day.

- Remind yourself of the commitment you made—and of how great you're going to feel as you make progress.

WEIGHT-LOSS BOOSTER

Read the Fine Print As you walk the aisles of your supermarket, it's tempting to just toss what you need into your cart and get out of the store as quickly as possible. But taking a little time to stop and read labels before you buy can have a big payoff: Women shoppers who read nutrition-facts panels weigh an average of 8.6 pounds less than those who simply grab and go.

BREAKFAST

Hunger Level

FOOD/AMOUNT _____

_____

_____

_____

_____

EMOTIONS _____

_____

_____

_____

LUNCH

Hunger Level

FOOD/AMOUNT _____

_____

_____

_____

_____

_____

_____

EMOTIONS _____

_____

_____

_____

_____

_____

DINNER

Hunger Level

FOOD/AMOUNT _____

_____

_____

_____

_____

_____

_____

EMOTIONS _____

_____

_____

_____

_____

_____

SNACK 1

Hunger Level

TIME/PLACE _____

FOOD/AMOUNT _____

EMOTIONS _____

SNACK 2

Hunger Level

TIME/PLACE _____

FOOD/AMOUNT _____

EMOTIONS _____

UNPLANNED EATING

Hunger Level

FOOD/AMOUNT _____

TIME/PLACE _____

EMOTIONS _____

DAILY MOVEMENT

Type of Activity	Minutes/Amount	How It Felt
AEROBIC Exercises:		
STRENGTHENING Exercises:		
FLEXIBILITY Exercises:		
BALANCE Exercises:		
INCIDENTAL MOVEMENT		

Junk Food-Junkie Alert

The Health-Conscious Chip Got a potato chip problem? Switch to kale chips that you make yourself. Here's how:

Preheat oven to 350°F. From one bunch (10 ounces) kale, remove and discard thick stems; tear leaves into large pieces. Spread leaves in single layer on 2 large cookie sheets. Spray leaves with nonstick cooking spray to coat lightly; sprinkle with salt. Bake 12 to 15 minutes or until kale chips are crisp but not browned. Cool on cookie sheets on wire racks.

DAILY ASSESSMENT

● Run an attitude check on yourself: Were you having any negative ("I'm angry at myself for eating that") or defeatist ("I don't have any willpower; I should just give up") thoughts today?

_____

_____

● Did you schedule in exercise and stick with it? If not, what changed your plans?

_____

_____

● Did you discover anything about food/movement/yourself today that you found helpful or motivating?

_____

_____

● What nice thing did you do for yourself today?

_____

_____

● Final thoughts on the day: Are you pleased with how the day went? What went well? What do you resolve to improve tomorrow?

_____

_____

_____

_____

_____

_____

✳ **DON'T FORGET**	*Check your to-do list before signing off for the night! It'll help you be ready for tomorrow.*

How Was Your Week?

If you had to describe your diet and exercise habits over the past seven days, how would you sum them up? It could be something like, "I am someone who eats healthy meals, but I still haven't conquered my late-night sweet tooth"; "I discovered that I'm a person who actually likes to walk"; or "I am someone who eats slowly and pays attention to what I'm consuming. Still can't make it to the gym." Write down your impressions, and then use them to set goals for next week.

_____

_____

_____

_____

_____

_____

_____

_____

_____

_____

GOALS FOR NEXT WEEK

_____

_____

_____

_____

_____

_____

_____

_____

_____

WEEK 3

WEEK 3

MEAL PLAN

DAY 1

Breakfast: New York Bagel
Lunch: Grilled Mozzarella &
Tomato Soup
Snack 1: PB & J–Inspired Yogurt
Dinner: Seared Salmon
with Sweet Potatoes
Snack 2: Ricotta-Fig Toasts

DAY 2

Breakfast: Peach Melba Yogurt
Lunch: Ham & Swiss
Snack 1: Hummus & Veggie Strips
Dinner: Basil-Orange Chicken
with Couscous
Snack 2: Chips & Cheese

DAY 3

Breakfast: Easy Oatmeal
Lunch: Cold Peanut Noodles
with Chicken
Snack 1: Iced-Coffee Break
Dinner: Two-Cheese Pita Pizzas with
Broccoli & Tomato
Snack 2: Cantaloupe Boat

DAY 4

Breakfast: Sunrise Soft Taco
Lunch: Microwavable Pasta Meal
Snack 1: Citrus Snack
Dinner: Chicken Parm Stacks
Snack 2: Out & About

DAY 5

Breakfast: Breakfast to Go
Lunch: Chicken Caesar Pitas
Snack 1: Strawberry Bagel Thin
Dinner: Niçoise Salad
Snack 2: Cocoa Fix

DAY 6

Breakfast:
Banana–Peanut Butter Smoothie
Lunch: Subway Sandwich & Soup
Snack 1: Cherries & Cheese
Dinner: Pomegranate-Glazed Salmon
Snack 2: Edamame Munchie

DAY 7

Breakfast: Breakfast Pizza
Lunch: Asian Chicken Salad
Snack 1: Honeydew "Sundae"
Dinner: Beef Ragu
Snack 2: Fruit & Grain Bar

Shopping List

For breakfasts, lunches, and dinners serving anywhere from one to six. Check recipes to make adjustments depending on the number of people you are feeding.

FRESH PRODUCE

- ¼ cup cilantro leaves
- 1 bunch mint
- ½ cup flat-leaf parsley leaves
- 3 green onions
- 20 grape tomatoes
- 2 plum tomatoes
- 6 medium regular tomatoes
- 8 cups sliced small head napa (Chinese) cabbage or shredded cabbage mix
- 1 head romaine lettuce
- 1 package (10 ounces) European-blend salad greens
- 2 packages (5 to 6 ounces each) baby spinach
- 8 ounces broccoli florets
- 1 large carrot
- 1 stalk celery
- ½ pound green beans
- 1 large red bell pepper
- 1 pound sweet potatoes
- 2 bunches radishes
- 1 pound yellow summer squash
- 2 packages (8 ounces each) stringless sugar snap peas
- 1 medium apple
- 3 bananas
- 1 small cantaloupe
- 10 cherries
- 18 grapes
- 1 pink grapefruit
- 1 honeydew melon
- 3 large oranges
- 2 peaches
- 1 pear
- ¼ cup pomegranate seeds
- ⅓ cup raspberries
- 3 large strawberries

SEAFOOD

- 8 pieces skinless center-cut salmon fillet (2½ pounds total)
- 1 ounce lox
- 1 can (5 ounces) no-salt-added albacore tuna

MEAT & POULTRY

- 1 pound lean ground beef
- 1 pound chicken-breast cutlets
- 8 skinless, boneless chicken-breast halves (3 pounds total)
- 1 pound shredded rotisserie chicken-breast meat
- 2 ounces lean lower-sodium ham

DAIRY

- 1 wedge Laughing Cow ⅓ Less Fat Classic Cream Cheese Spread
- ¾ ounce aged goat cheese or Brie
- ½ cup crumbled goat cheese
- 2 tablespoons shredded reduced-fat Monterey Jack cheese
- 1½ ounces part-skim mozzarella cheese
- 1 stick part-skim mozzarella string cheese
- 1 slice reduced-fat Swiss cheese
- ½ cup low-fat (1%), low-sodium cottage cheese

GRAIN PRODUCTS

- 1 cup whole wheat couscous
- 4 ounces whole wheat linguine or spaghetti
- 1 package (13¼ ounces) whole-grain penne pasta

FROZEN FOODS

1 Healthy Choice Italian Sausage Pasta Bake meal

1 bag (16 ounces) shelled edamame

CANNED GOODS

2 cans (15 ounces each) no-salt-added garbanzo beans (chickpeas)

1 can (19 ounces) white kidney (cannellini) beans

¼ cup marinara sauce

1 cup Campbell's 100% Natural Harvest Tomato with Basil Soup

1 can (14½ ounces) no-salt-added fire-roasted diced tomatoes

MISCELLANEOUS

24 Emerald Cocoa Roast Almonds (dark-chocolate flavor) or Planters Smoked Almonds

5 dried-apricot halves

1 Kashi Chewy Cherry Dark Chocolate Granola Bar

1 Kind Mini Fruit & Nut Delight Bar

1 Kind Nuts & Spices Bar in Madagascar Vanilla Almond

¼ cup hummus

6 slices whole-grain melba toast

½ cup Kalamata or large black olives

½ cup orange juice

¾ cup no-sugar-added 100% pomegranate juice

1 can (11½ ounces) low-sodium tomato or vegetable juice

5 Food Should Taste Good Multigrain tortilla chips

DAY 1

TO-DO LIST

- Reread your pledge.

- Assess your schedule for today. Is anything going to make it difficult to stick to your diet? Strategize to overcome obstacles.

- Put some formal exercise on today's calendar or think about ways you can move your body.

- Plan for tomorrow's meals tonight. What are you going to eat? Do you have everything you need? If you're brown-bagging tomorrow's lunch, save time by assembling what you can now.

- Pack your journal or make sure you have a pen and paper (or a smartphone) for making notes throughout the day.

- Remind yourself of the commitment you made—and of how great you're going to feel as you make progress.

MINDLESS-MUNCHER ALERT

Tactical Snacking If you usually end up downing a whole box of crackers or bag of chips, you may be less likely to overdo it if you eat treats with protein or produce. Try crackers with a low-fat hummus dip or a yogurt-dill mix. Put a few chips on a plate and team them with carrot or celery sticks. If you've got a sweet tooth, have a square of dark chocolate with some berries.

BREAKFAST

Hunger Level

FOOD/AMOUNT _____

_____

_____

_____

_____

EMOTIONS _____

_____

_____

_____

_____

LUNCH

Hunger Level

FOOD/AMOUNT _____

_____

_____

_____

_____

EMOTIONS _____

_____

_____

_____

_____

DINNER

Hunger Level

FOOD/AMOUNT _____

_____

_____

_____

_____

EMOTIONS _____

_____

_____

_____

SNACK 1

Hunger Level

TIME/PLACE _____

FOOD/AMOUNT _____

EMOTIONS _____

SNACK 2

Hunger Level

TIME/PLACE _____

FOOD/AMOUNT _____

EMOTIONS _____

UNPLANNED EATING

Hunger Level

FOOD/AMOUNT _____

TIME/PLACE _____

EMOTIONS _____

DAILY MOVEMENT

Type of Activity	Minutes/Amount	How It Felt
AEROBIC Exercises:		
STRENGTHENING Exercises:		
FLEXIBILITY Exercises:		
BALANCE Exercises:		
INCIDENTAL MOVEMENT		

Motivation Tips From the Trenches

How do GH readers and staffers stay motivated to exercise?

"The scale next to my bed is my number one motivator."
—*Aileen Raymundo, GH Facebook friend*

"Realizing that I can't self-motivate on a treadmill or elliptical machine, but I love taking classes, has helped me make it to the gym on a more regular basis."
—*Cathy Lo, GH associate food editor*

DAILY ASSESSMENT

- What changes are you beginning to notice? Have you dropped as many pounds as you hoped you would? If not, think about possible reasons why. Do you see improvements in your skin and your energy level? Be sure to write down your triumphs and frustrations.

- Did anything unexpected occur today? How did you cope? If you didn't cope well, how would you handle it in the future?

- Did you schedule in exercise and stick with it? If not, what changed your plans?

- Did you discover anything about food/movement/yourself today that you found helpful or motivating?

- What nice thing did you do for yourself today?

- Final thoughts on the day: Are you pleased with how the day went? What went well? What do you resolve to change tomorrow?

* **DON'T FORGET** | *Check your to-do list before signing off for the night! It'll help you be ready for tomorrow.*

TO-DO LIST

- Assess your schedule for today. Is anything going to make it difficult to stick to your diet? Strategize to overcome obstacles.

- Put some formal exercise on today's calendar or think about extra ways you can move your body.

- Plan for tomorrow's meals tonight. What are you going to eat? Do you have everything you need? If you're brown-bagging tomorrow's lunch, save time by assembling what you can now.

- Pack your journal or make sure you have a pen and paper (or a smartphone) for making notes throughout the day.

- Remind yourself of the commitment you made—and of how great you're going to feel as you make progress.

LIQUID-CALORIE-LOVER ALERT

Rethink Your Drink Sodas may be fizzy and fruit punch may seem festive, but apparently they don't confer those happy attributes to those who drink them. After tracking 264,000 adults, National Institutes of Health researchers found that fruit-punch drinkers and those who drank more than four cans of regular soda per day were 38% and 30%, respectively, more likely to develop depression than non-pop-drinkers. Diet soft drinks were also associated with the blues.

BREAKFAST

Hunger Level

FOOD/AMOUNT _____

_____
_____
_____
_____
_____

EMOTIONS _____

_____
_____
_____
_____

LUNCH

Hunger Level

FOOD/AMOUNT _____

_____

_____

_____

_____

_____

_____

EMOTIONS _____

_____

_____

_____

_____

_____

DINNER

Hunger Level

FOOD/AMOUNT _____

_____

_____

_____

_____

_____

_____

EMOTIONS _____

_____

_____

_____

_____

_____

SNACK 1

Hunger Level

TIME/PLACE _____

FOOD/AMOUNT _____

EMOTIONS _____

SNACK 2

Hunger Level

TIME/PLACE _____

FOOD/AMOUNT _____

EMOTIONS _____

UNPLANNED EATING

Hunger Level

FOOD/AMOUNT _____

TIME/PLACE _____

EMOTIONS _____

DAILY MOVEMENT

Type of Activity	Minutes/Amount	How It Felt
AEROBIC Exercises:		
STRENGTHENING Exercises:		
FLEXIBILITY Exercises:		
BALANCE Exercises:		
INCIDENTAL MOVEMENT		

Bone Builders When it comes to thwarting bone loss that occurs with aging, all workouts are not created equal. Your best osteoporosis preventers:

- **Strength training** stimulates the growth of new bone via muscles tugging on bones. Exercise bands, calisthenics, and weight-lifting exercises all do the trick.

- **Cardiovascular workouts** build bone if they are weight-bearing. Brisk walking, jogging, aerobic dance, jumping rope, stair climbing, and hiking all qualify.

- **Sports,** like weight-bearing cardio, offer fracture protection. Good choices: racquet sports, soccer, volleyball, and basketball.

DAILY ASSESSMENT

- Did anything unexpected occur today? How did you cope? If you didn't cope well, how would you handle it in the future?

_____

_____

- Did you schedule in exercise and stick with it? If not, what changed your plans?

_____

_____

- Did you discover anything about food/movement/yourself today that you found helpful or motivating?

_____

_____

- What nice thing did you do for yourself today?

_____

_____

- Final thoughts on the day: Are you pleased with how the day went? What went well? What do you resolve to improve tomorrow?

_____

_____

_____

_____

_____

| ✻ **DON'T FORGET** | _Check your to-do list before signing off for the night! It'll help you be ready for tomorrow._ |

TO-DO LIST

- Assess your schedule for today. Is anything going to make it difficult to stick to your diet? Strategize to overcome obstacles.

- Put some formal exercise on today's calendar or think about extra ways you can move your body.

- Plan for tomorrow's meals tonight. What are you going to eat? Do you have everything you need? If you're brown-bagging tomorrow's lunch, save time by assembling what you can now.

- Pack your journal or make sure you have a pen and paper (or a smartphone) for making notes throughout the day.

- Remind yourself of the commitment you made—and of how great you're going to feel as you make progress.

CRAVINGS CONTROL

Water Works When researchers at Stanford University analyzed the diets of 173 overweight women, they found that those who consumed six glasses of water a day took in 200 fewer calories than their less hydrated peers. Another study found that people who drank two glasses of water before meals lost 41% more weight than those who didn't. Drink up!

BREAKFAST

Hunger Level

FOOD/AMOUNT _____

EMOTIONS _____

LUNCH

Hunger Level

FOOD/AMOUNT _____

_____
_____
_____
_____
_____
_____
_____

EMOTIONS _____

_____
_____
_____
_____
_____

DINNER

Hunger Level

FOOD/AMOUNT _____

_____
_____
_____
_____
_____
_____
_____

EMOTIONS _____

_____
_____
_____
_____
_____

SNACK 1

*Hunger
Level*

TIME/PLACE _____

FOOD/AMOUNT _____

EMOTIONS _____

SNACK 2

*Hunger
Level*

TIME/PLACE _____

FOOD/AMOUNT _____

EMOTIONS _____

UNPLANNED EATING

*Hunger
Level*

FOOD/AMOUNT _____

TIME/PLACE _____

EMOTIONS _____

DAILY MOVEMENT

Type of Activity	Minutes/Amount	How It Felt
AEROBIC Exercises:		
STRENGTHENING Exercises:		
FLEXIBILITY Exercises:		
BALANCE Exercises:		
INCIDENTAL MOVEMENT		

Sugar's Not-So-Sweet Effect Sugar and other refined carbohydrates create reactions in the body that increase production of AGEs—advanced glycation end products. These compounds can interfere with repair of collagen and elastin in the skin and expose cells in the body to more oxidative stress and inflammation. Be on the lookout for sugar's aliases on packaged-food ingredient lists: glucose, fructose, maltose, high-fructose corn syrup, brown rice syrup, evaporated cane juice, cane crystals, agave, fruit-juice concentrate, honey, and molasses.

DAILY ASSESSMENT

- Did anything unexpected occur today? How did you cope? If you didn't cope well, how would you handle it in the future?

_____

_____

- Did you schedule in exercise and stick with it? If not, what changed your plans?

_____

_____

- Did you discover anything about food/movement/yourself today that you found helpful or motivating?

_____

_____

- What nice thing did you do for yourself today?

_____

_____

- Final thoughts on the day: Are you pleased with how the day went? What went well? What do you resolve to improve tomorrow?

_____

_____

_____

_____

_____

_____

_____

---

* DON'T FORGET | _Check your to-do list before signing off for the night!_
It'll help you be ready for tomorrow.

TO-DO LIST

- Assess your schedule for today. Is anything going to make it difficult to stick to your diet? Strategize to overcome obstacles.

- Put some formal exercise on today's calendar or think about extra ways you can move your body.

- Plan for tomorrow's meals tonight. What are you going to eat? Do you have everything you need? If you're brown-bagging tomorrow's lunch, save time by assembling what you can now.

- Pack your journal or make sure you have a pen and paper (or a smartphone) for making notes throughout the day.

- Remind yourself of the commitment you made—and of how great you're going to feel as you make progress.

MOVE MORE, LOSE MORE

A Super Calorie Burner If you haven't tried Zumba, the dance-based aerobic workout everyone's talking about, maybe you should give it a shot. A University of Wisconsin-La Crosse study found that a 40-minute Zumba class torches an average of 370 calories!

BREAKFAST

Hunger Level

FOOD/AMOUNT _____

_____

_____

_____

_____

_____

EMOTIONS _____

_____

_____

_____

_____

LUNCH

Hunger Level

FOOD/AMOUNT _____

_____
_____
_____
_____
_____
_____

EMOTIONS _____

_____
_____
_____
_____

DINNER

Hunger Level

FOOD/AMOUNT _____

_____
_____
_____
_____
_____
_____

EMOTIONS _____

_____
_____
_____
_____

SNACK 1

Hunger Level

TIME/PLACE _____

FOOD/AMOUNT _____

EMOTIONS _____

SNACK 2

Hunger Level

TIME/PLACE _____

FOOD/AMOUNT _____

EMOTIONS _____

UNPLANNED EATING

Hunger Level

FOOD/AMOUNT _____

TIME/PLACE _____

EMOTIONS _____

DAILY MOVEMENT

Type of Activity	Minutes/Amount	How It Felt
AEROBIC Exercises:		
STRENGTHENING Exercises:		
FLEXIBILITY Exercises:		
BALANCE Exercises:		
INCIDENTAL MOVEMENT		

Diet Phraseology What's in a word? A lot, as it turns out. Saying "I don't" instead of "I can't" when there's a slice of chocolate cake staring you in the face may increase your ability to say no. "'Can't' signals deprivation, while 'don't' helps you feel determined," explains Vanessa Patrick, Ph.D., who has researched swapping the terms. Saying "I don't eat chips and guacamole" rather than "I can't eat chips and guacamole" when you're out with friends may also ease social pressure, helping your buddies get clued in to the strength of your conviction to eat healthfully.

DAILY ASSESSMENT

- Did anything unexpected occur today? How did you cope? If you didn't cope well, how would you handle it in the future?

_____

_____

- Did you schedule in exercise and stick with it? If not, what changed your plans?

_____

_____

- Did you discover anything about food/movement/yourself today that you found helpful or motivating?

_____

_____

- What nice thing did you do for yourself today?

_____

_____

- Final thoughts on the day: Are you pleased with how the day went? What went well? What do you resolve to improve tomorrow?

_____

_____

_____

_____

_____

_____

✻ DON'T FORGET | _Check your to-do list before signing off for the night! It'll help you be ready for tomorrow._

DAY 5

TO-DO LIST

- Assess your schedule for today. Is anything going to make it difficult to stick to your diet? Strategize to overcome obstacles.

- Put some formal exercise on today's calendar or think about extra ways you can move your body.

- Plan for tomorrow's meals tonight. What are you going to eat? Do you have everything you need? If you're brown-bagging tomorrow's lunch, save time by assembling what you can now.

- Pack your journal or make sure you have a pen and paper (or a smartphone) for making notes throughout the day.

- Remind yourself of the commitment you made—and of how great you're going to feel as you make progress.

MORE MINDFUL EATING

Go Ahead, Ruin Your Dinner We know your mother always told you not to do it, but now that you're a grown-up, go ahead and have a snack before dinner. Neil Fredman, one of our diet testers, got into the habit of eating an apple about a half hour before his evening meal. "That time lapse makes a difference," he says. "I didn't sit down for dinner feeling famished."

BREAKFAST

Hunger Level

FOOD/AMOUNT _____

_____
_____
_____
_____

EMOTIONS _____

_____
_____
_____
_____

LUNCH

Hunger Level

FOOD/AMOUNT _____

_____
_____
_____
_____

EMOTIONS _____

_____
_____
_____
_____

TESTER TIP

**"I've spread my meals out to 10:30ish and
2:30ish because I usually don't eat
in the mornings. That way I'm not starving
when I walk in the door at 5."**

—Leigh Gillam, 12 pounds and 5 inches lost

DINNER

Hunger Level

FOOD/AMOUNT _____

_____
_____
_____
_____

EMOTIONS _____

_____
_____
_____
_____

SNACK 1

Hunger Level

TIME/PLACE _____

FOOD/AMOUNT _____

EMOTIONS _____

SNACK 2

Hunger Level

TIME/PLACE _____

FOOD/AMOUNT _____

EMOTIONS _____

UNPLANNED EATING

Hunger Level

FOOD/AMOUNT _____

TIME/PLACE _____

EMOTIONS _____

DAILY MOVEMENT

Type of Activity	Minutes/Amount	How It Felt
AEROBIC Exercises:		
STRENGTHENING Exercises:		
FLEXIBILITY Exercises:		
BALANCE Exercises:		
INCIDENTAL MOVEMENT		

Build a Better Picnic Alfresco dining can be a fat-laden feast—or a simply delightful calorie-conscious spread. Here are the best picnic picks.

INSTEAD OF...	CHOOSE	CALORIES SAVED
1 cup of lemonade	1 cup of sparkling water with a lemon wedge	109
1 fried chicken breast	1 grilled, skinless breast	255
1/2 cup of mayo-based potato salad	1/2 cup of coleslaw	132
1/2 cup chocolate ice cream from the truck	3 chocolate-covered strawberries	126

DAILY ASSESSMENT

● Did anything unexpected occur today? How did you cope? If you didn't cope well, how would you handle it in the future?

_____

_____

● Did you schedule in exercise and stick with it? If not, what changed your plans?

_____

_____

● Did you discover anything about food/movement/yourself today that you found helpful or motivating?

_____

_____

● What nice thing did you do for yourself today?

_____

_____

● Final thoughts on the day: Are you pleased with how the day went? What went well? What do you resolve to improve tomorrow?

_____

_____

✳ DON'T FORGET	*Check your to-do list before signing off for the night! It'll help you be ready for tomorrow.*

TO-DO LIST

- Assess your schedule for today. Is anything going to make it difficult to stick to your diet? Strategize to overcome obstacles.

- Put some formal exercise on today's calendar or think about extra ways you can move your body.

- Plan for tomorrow's meals tonight. What are you going to eat? Do you have everything you need? If you're brown-bagging tomorrow's lunch, save time by assembling what you can now.

- Pack your journal or make sure you have a pen and paper (or a smartphone) for making notes throughout the day.

- Remind yourself of the commitment you made—and of how great you're going to feel as you make progress.

ANTI-AGING EATING

Dewier Skin Lutein—now, that's not a nutrient you hear much about. It should be on your radar, though, if you're hoping to avoid dry, old-looking skin. Lutein helps keep your complexion hydrated and also protects your eyes from sun damage. Eggs, leafy greens, broccoli, corn, and peas—all amply available in the 7 Years Younger Meal Plan—are the best sources.

BREAKFAST

Hunger Level

FOOD/AMOUNT _____

_____

_____

_____

_____

_____

EMOTIONS _____

_____

_____

_____

_____

LUNCH

Hunger Level

FOOD/AMOUNT _____

_____
_____
_____
_____
_____
_____
_____

EMOTIONS _____

_____
_____
_____
_____
_____
_____

DINNER

Hunger Level

FOOD/AMOUNT _____

_____
_____
_____
_____
_____
_____
_____

EMOTIONS _____

_____
_____
_____
_____
_____
_____

SNACK 1

Hunger Level

TIME/PLACE _____

FOOD/AMOUNT _____

EMOTIONS _____

SNACK 2

Hunger Level

TIME/PLACE _____

FOOD/AMOUNT _____

EMOTIONS _____

UNPLANNED EATING

Hunger Level

FOOD/AMOUNT _____

TIME/PLACE _____

EMOTIONS _____

DAILY MOVEMENT

Type of Activity	Minutes/Amount	How It Felt
AEROBIC Exercises:		
STRENGTHENING Exercises:		
FLEXIBILITY Exercises:		
BALANCE Exercises:		
INCIDENTAL MOVEMENT		

Walking It Off Most of us can look at a calorie count and make a judgment: high, low, or just right. But what if a food's impact were noted in more practical terms? Researchers at Texas Christian University had diners order from restaurant menus that listed the amount of brisk walking it would take to work off each dish. The dose of reality worked: The diners were less likely to overeat when they used these menus than when they used menus listing only calories. Here's a little reality check:

FOOD TO BURN OFF	BRISK WALKING REQUIRED
1 slice pizza *(304 cals.)*	**52 minutes**
½ cup premium vanilla ice cream *(250 cals.)*	**43 minutes**
1 medium chocolate donut *(194 cals.)*	**33 minutes**
2 chocolate chip cookies *(160 cals.)*	**28 minutes**
1-ounce bag of potato chips *(154 cals.)*	**27 minutes**

Calories burned based on a 140-pound woman.

DAILY ASSESSMENT

● Did anything unexpected occur today? How did you cope? If you didn't cope well, how would you handle it in the future?

● Did you schedule in exercise and stick with it? If not, what changed your plans?

● Did you discover anything about food/movement/yourself today that you found helpful or motivating?

● What nice thing did you do for yourself today?

● Final thoughts on the day: Are you pleased with how the day went? What went well? What do you resolve to improve tomorrow?

✳ **DON'T FORGET** | *Check your to-do list before signing off for the night! It'll help you be ready for tomorrow.*

DAY 7

TO-DO LIST

- Assess your schedule for today. Is anything going to make it difficult to stick to your diet? Strategize to overcome obstacles.

- Put some formal exercise on today's calendar or think about extra ways you can move your body.

- Plan for tomorrow's meals tonight. What are you going to eat? Do you have everything you need? If you're brown-bagging tomorrow's lunch, save time by assembling what you can now.

- Pack your journal or make sure you have a pen and paper (or a smartphone) for making notes throughout the day.

- Remind yourself of the commitment you made—and of how great you're going to feel as you make progress.

MEAL-SKIPPER ALERT

Ease Into Your Morning Meal Research suggests that A.M. meal skippers tend to take in more calories in the evening. If you're not hungry when the alarm rings, have at least half of your breakfast calories within three hours of waking, then the other half as a mid-morning snack. This may help you slowly break the cycle of eating most of your calories at day's end.

BREAKFAST

Hunger Level

FOOD/AMOUNT _____

EMOTIONS _____

LUNCH

Hunger Level

FOOD/AMOUNT _____

_____

_____

_____

_____

_____

_____

_____

EMOTIONS _____

_____

_____

_____

_____

_____

DINNER

Hunger Level

FOOD/AMOUNT _____

_____

_____

_____

_____

_____

_____

_____

EMOTIONS _____

_____

_____

_____

_____

_____

SNACK 1

Hunger Level

TIME/PLACE _____

FOOD/AMOUNT _____

EMOTIONS _____

SNACK 2

Hunger Level

TIME/PLACE _____

FOOD/AMOUNT _____

EMOTIONS _____

UNPLANNED EATING

Hunger Level

FOOD/AMOUNT _____

TIME/PLACE _____

EMOTIONS _____

DAILY MOVEMENT

Type of Activity	Minutes/Amount	How It Felt
AEROBIC Exercises:		
STRENGTHENING Exercises:		
FLEXIBILITY Exercises:		
BALANCE Exercises:		
INCIDENTAL MOVEMENT		

Build a Better Popcorn Rich in fiber and antioxidants, popcorn is a great anti-aging snack—if you make it yourself (a small bag of movie popcorn can have 400-plus calories!). Microwave a 94%-fat-free popcorn, or cook popcorn on the stovetop using a small amount of oil (1 tablespoon of heart-healthy canola oil per ½ cup of kernels). Then, for added flavor, try one of these mix-ins:

- **2 teaspoons chili powder, 1 teaspoon cumin**
- **2 teaspoons smoked paprika**
- **3 tablespoons grated Parmesan cheese, ¼ teaspoon garlic**

DAILY ASSESSMENT

- Did anything unexpected occur today? How did you cope? If you didn't cope well, how would you handle it in the future?

_____

_____

- Did you schedule in exercise and stick with it? If not, what changed your plans?

_____

_____

- Did you discover anything about food/movement/yourself today that you found helpful or motivating?

_____

_____

- What nice thing did you do for yourself today?

_____

_____

- Final thoughts on the day: Are you pleased with how the day went? What went well? What do you resolve to improve tomorrow?

_____

_____

_____

_____

_____

| ✻ **DON'T FORGET** | *Check your to-do list before signing off for the night! It'll help you be ready for tomorrow.* |

How Was Your Week?

Now is a good time to assess whether or not you're getting the support you need. How are your family, friends, and colleagues handling the changes you've made these past few weeks? Are they being helpful and understanding? If they are, write about the gratitude you feel for their cheerleading and assistance. If not, contemplate how you can ask them to be more supportive or, if the support seems too elusive, write about why you're determined to succeed even without help.

_____

_____

_____

_____

_____

_____

_____

_____

_____

_____

_____

GOALS FOR NEXT WEEK

_____

_____

_____

_____

_____

_____

_____

_____

_____

_____

WEEK 4

WEEK 4

DAY 1
Breakfast: Huevos Rancheros
Lunch: Open-Face Jarlsberg
Sandwich with Greens
Snack 1: Blueberry Lassi
Dinner: Orange Pork & Asparagus
Stir-Fry
Snack 2: Pistachios

DAY 2
Breakfast: Easy Oatmeal
Lunch: Chinese Rice Bowl
Snack 1: Prosciutto & Mozzarella Plate
Dinner: Lemon-Mint
Chicken Cutlets on Watercress
Snack 2: Cheese Bite

DAY 3
Breakfast: Strawberry Cereal
Lunch: Chipotle Lunch
Snack 1: Hummus & Veggie Strips
Dinner: Garden-Vegetable Omelet
Snack 2: Pudding Parfait

DAY 4
Breakfast: Sweet Stuffed Waffle
Lunch: Greek Feast
Snack 1: Iced-Coffee Break
Dinner: Crispy Fish Sandwiches
Snack 2: Movie Mix

DAY 5
Breakfast: Smoked-Salmon
Scrambled Eggs
Lunch: Mexican Chicken Salad
Snack 1: Pineapple Plate
Dinner: Ziti with Peas,
Grape Tomatoes & Ricotta
Snack 2: Chips & Cheese

DAY 6
Breakfast: Grab & Go
Lunch: Grilled Mozzarella &
Tomato Soup
Snack 1: Veggies & Dill Dip
Dinner: Chicken & Veggie Stir-Fry
Snack 2: Ricotta-Fig Toasts

DAY 7
Breakfast:
California Breakfast Bruschetta
Lunch: Jambalaya
Snack 1: Yogurt Sundae
Dinner: Fresh Salmon Burgers with
Capers and Dill
Snack 2: Cantaloupe Boat

Shopping List

For breakfasts, lunches, and dinners serving anywhere from one to six. Check recipes to make adjustments depending on the number of people you are feeding.

FRESH PRODUCE

- ¼ cup basil leaves
- 1 small bunch chives
- ¼ cup cilantro leaves
- ½ cup dill
- ½ cup mint leaves
- 1 tablespoon oregano leaves
- ½ cup flat-leaf parsley leaves
- 7 green onions
- 2 pints (12 ounces each) grape or cherry tomatoes
- 4 plum tomatoes
- 1 regular tomato
- 3 cups baby arugula
- 3 cups shredded red cabbage
- 1 large head romaine or green leaf lettuce
- 1 bag (5 to 6 ounces) baby spinach
- 1 bag (4 ounces) baby watercress
- 1½ pounds thin asparagus
- 12 baby carrots
- 2 cups shredded carrots
- 2 seedless (English) cucumbers
- 2 green bell peppers
- 4 red bell peppers
- 1 large yellow bell pepper
- 8 ounces red potatoes
- 1 small and 4 medium zucchini
- 1 avocado
- 1 small and 1 medium apple
- 1 banana
- 1 pint (12 ounces) blackberries
- 1 cantaloupe
- 1 wedge honeydew melon
- 1 kiwifruit
- 3 oranges
- ½ cup pineapple chunks
- 2 teaspoons pomegranate seeds
- 5 raspberries
- 5 strawberries

SEAFOOD

- 4 skinless flounder fillets (1 pound total)
- 1 pound skin-on salmon fillets
- 5 ounces thinly sliced smoked salmon

MEAT & POULTRY

- 2½ pounds skinless, boneless chicken-breast halves
- ¾ pound pork tenderloin
- ½ cup shredded cooked chicken-breast meat
- ½ ounce very thinly sliced prosciutto
- 1 link precooked garlic chicken sausage

DAIRY

- 1 Mini Babybel Sharp Original or Gouda cheese
- 2 teaspoons crumbled blue cheese
- 1 tablespoon Philadelphia ⅓ Less Fat Chive & Onion Cream Cheese
- 4 ounces reduced-fat feta cheese
- 6 ounces Jarlsberg cheese
- 2½ ounces part-skim mozzarella cheese
- 1 stick part-skim mozzarella string cheese
- 1 container (3½ ounces) Chobani Bites Raspberry with Dark Chocolate Chips
- ½ cup low-fat (1%), low-sodium cottage cheese
- 1 container (6 ounces) sugar-free vanilla pudding
- 3 tablespoons tzatziki sauce

GRAIN PRODUCTS

¾ cup whole wheat couscous

14 ounces whole-grain ziti pasta

2 containers (4.4 ounces each) Minute Ready to Serve brown rice

2 packages (8.8 ounces each) precooked or Uncle Ben's Ready Rice brown rice

FROZEN FOODS

2 Van's 8 Whole Grains waffles

¼ cup frozen blueberries

1½ cups shelled edamame

2 cups frozen peas

CANNED GOODS

2 cans (15 ounces each) black beans

1 can (15 ounces) garbanzo beans (chickpeas)

1 cup Campbell's 100% Natural Harvest Tomato with Basil Soup

1 can (28 ounces) whole peeled tomatoes in juice

MISCELLANEOUS

8 roasted cashews or dry-roasted peanuts

½ cup hummus

½ cup Edy's/Dreyer's Slow Churned No Sugar Added Ice Cream, vanilla or Neapolitan flavor

2 slices whole-grain melba toast

1 cup Good Health Half Naked Popcorn

1 can (11½ ounces) low-sodium tomato or vegetable juice

15 Food Should Taste Good Multigrain tortilla chips

TO-DO LIST

- Reread your pledge.

- Assess your schedule for today. Is anything going to make it difficult to stick to your diet? Strategize to overcome obstacles.

- Put some formal exercise on today's calendar or think about ways you can move your body.

- Plan for tomorrow's meals tonight. What are you going to eat? Do you have everything you need? If you're brown-bagging tomorrow's lunch, save time by assembling what you can now.

- Pack your journal or make sure you have a pen and paper (or a smartphone) for making notes throughout the day.

- Remind yourself of the commitment you made—and of how great you're going to feel as you make progress.

MINDLESS-MUNCHER ALERT

Set the Mood Dining in a soothing space helped restaurant-goers eat 18% less in a recent study. To mimic the effect at home:

- Turn off the TV and lower the lights to make the setting more relaxed. That'll help you eat more slowly and allow fullness signals to register in your brain.
- Put on some mellow tunes. Leisurely music will reduce your fork-to-mouth pace.

BREAKFAST

Hunger Level

FOOD/AMOUNT _____

EMOTIONS _____

LUNCH

Hunger
Level

FOOD/AMOUNT _____

_____

_____

_____

_____

EMOTIONS _____

_____

_____

_____

_____

TESTER TIP

"The best thing about this plan is the strategic nature of the eating. It's not just about 'eating less'; it's about eating the right stuff at the right time."

—*Carol Scudder-Danilowicz, 8½ pounds and 4¾ inches lost*

DINNER

Hunger
Level

FOOD/AMOUNT _____

_____

_____

_____

_____

EMOTIONS _____

_____

_____

_____

_____

SNACK 1

Hunger Level

TIME/PLACE _____

FOOD/AMOUNT _____

EMOTIONS _____

SNACK 2

Hunger Level

TIME/PLACE _____

FOOD/AMOUNT _____

EMOTIONS _____

UNPLANNED EATING

Hunger Level

FOOD/AMOUNT _____

TIME/PLACE _____

EMOTIONS _____

DAILY MOVEMENT

Type of Activity	Minutes/Amount	How It Felt
AEROBIC Exercises:		
STRENGTHENING Exercises:		
FLEXIBILITY Exercises:		
BALANCE Exercises:		
INCIDENTAL MOVEMENT		

Stick-To-It Strategy

Motivation Tips From the Trenches
How do GH readers stay motivated to exercise?

"I walk my kids to the bus stop and then run home. That gives me enough of a boost to use the home gym or go for a bike ride."
—*Polly Vee, GH Facebook friend*

"When I start the day off by eating a healthy meal, I crave 'good' food for the rest of the day."
—*Jennifer Moreno, GH Facebook friend*

DAILY ASSESSMENT

● What seemed difficult at first that's easy now? Or what seemed easy at first that's challenging you now?

_____

● Did anything unexpected occur today? How did you cope? If you didn't cope well, how would you handle it in the future?

_____

● Did you schedule in exercise and follow through? If not, what changed your plans?

_____

● Did you discover anything about food/movement/yourself today that you found helpful or motivating?

_____

● What nice thing did you do for yourself today?

_____

● Final thoughts on the day: Are you pleased with how the day went? What went well? What do you resolve to change tomorrow?

_____

_____

_____

✳ **DON'T FORGET**	*Check your to-do list before signing off for the night! It'll help you be ready for tomorrow.*

DAY 2

TO-DO LIST

- Assess your schedule for today. Is anything going to make it difficult to stick to your diet? Strategize to overcome obstacles.

- Put some formal exercise on today's calendar or think about extra ways you can move your body.

- Plan for tomorrow's meals tonight. What are you going to eat? Do you have everything you need? If you're brown-bagging tomorrow's lunch, save time by assembling what you can now.

- Pack your journal or make sure you have a pen and paper (or a smartphone) for making notes throughout the day.

- Remind yourself of the commitment you made—and of how great you're going to feel as you make progress.

MOVE MORE, LOSE MORE

Short Bouts Count If you can't fit in a 20-minute walk, simply break it up— the cumulative time will count toward calorie-burning and health benefits. For best results, aim to get in two to three 10-minute walks at least four days a week. Adding in hills and speed intervals will help you get even more out of those 10 minutes. What's most important, though, is building an exercise habit.

BREAKFAST

Hunger Level

FOOD/AMOUNT _____

_____

_____

_____

_____

_____

EMOTIONS _____

_____

_____

_____

_____

LUNCH

*Hunger
Level*

FOOD/AMOUNT _____

_____
_____
_____
_____
_____
_____
_____

EMOTIONS _____

_____
_____
_____
_____
_____

DINNER

*Hunger
Level*

FOOD/AMOUNT _____

_____
_____
_____
_____
_____
_____

EMOTIONS _____

_____
_____
_____
_____
_____

SNACK 1

TIME/PLACE _____ *Hunger Level*

FOOD/AMOUNT _____

EMOTIONS _____

SNACK 2

TIME/PLACE _____ *Hunger Level*

FOOD/AMOUNT _____

EMOTIONS _____

UNPLANNED EATING

FOOD/AMOUNT _____ *Hunger Level*

TIME/PLACE _____

EMOTIONS _____

DAILY MOVEMENT

Type of Activity	Minutes/Amount	How It Felt
AEROBIC Exercises:		
STRENGTHENING Exercises:		
FLEXIBILITY Exercises:		
BALANCE Exercises:		
INCIDENTAL MOVEMENT		

Liquid-Calorie-Lover Alert

Cure for the Water Blahs Some people find water refreshing; others find it utterly boring. If you fall into the latter camp, consider a few ways to jazz it up.

- Add a sprig of fresh mint or a slice of lemon, lime, or orange for flavor
- Add cucumber slices to a pitcher of water, then aim to finish the pitcher by day's end
- Purchase no-calorie flavored waters
- Opt for sparkling water, seltzer, or club soda—fizz can trick your tummy into thinking it's full

DAILY ASSESSMENT

- Did anything unexpected occur today? How did you cope? If you didn't cope well, how would you handle it in the future?

- Did you schedule in exercise and stick with it? If not, what changed your plans?

- Did you discover anything about food/movement/yourself today that you found helpful or motivating?

- What nice thing did you do for yourself today?

- Final thoughts on the day: Are you pleased with how the day went? What went well? What do you resolve to improve tomorrow?

✻ DON'T FORGET | *Check your to-do list before signing off for the night! It'll help you be ready for tomorrow.*

DAY 3

TO-DO LIST

- Assess your schedule for today. Is anything going to make it difficult to stick to your diet? Strategize to overcome obstacles.

- Put some formal exercise on today's calendar or think about extra ways you can move your body.

- Plan for tomorrow's meals tonight. What are you going to eat? Do you have everything you need? If you're brown-bagging tomorrow's lunch, save time by assembling what you can now.

- Pack your journal or make sure you have a pen and paper (or a smartphone) for making notes throughout the day.

- Remind yourself of the commitment you made—and of how great you're going to feel as you make progress.

ANTI-AGING EATING

Protein Plus This diet calls for a little more protein than the USDA standards. In addition to helping prevent hunger, protein is key for bone strength as you age. As part of the Framingham Osteoporosis Study, researchers looked at the protein intake of more than 900 men and women, average age 75; those who ate the most had a lower risk of hip fracture.

BREAKFAST

Hunger Level

FOOD/AMOUNT _____

_____

_____

_____

_____

_____

EMOTIONS _____

_____

_____

_____

_____

LUNCH

Hunger Level

FOOD/AMOUNT _____

_____

_____

_____

_____

_____

_____

_____

EMOTIONS _____

_____

_____

_____

_____

_____

DINNER

Hunger Level

FOOD/AMOUNT _____

_____

_____

_____

_____

_____

_____

_____

EMOTIONS _____

_____

_____

_____

_____

_____

SNACK 1

Hunger Level

TIME/PLACE _____

FOOD/AMOUNT _____

EMOTIONS _____

SNACK 2

Hunger Level

TIME/PLACE _____

FOOD/AMOUNT _____

EMOTIONS _____

UNPLANNED EATING

Hunger Level

FOOD/AMOUNT _____

TIME/PLACE _____

EMOTIONS _____

DAILY MOVEMENT

Type of Activity	Minutes/Amount	How It Felt
AEROBIC Exercises:		
STRENGTHENING Exercises:		
FLEXIBILITY Exercises:		
BALANCE Exercises:		
INCIDENTAL MOVEMENT		

Meal-Skipper Alert

Clever Convenience Foods By now you know you're more likely to reach for the wrong food when you don't have the right stuff on hand. That's a particular hazard when you're on the run, but if you stockpile these smart snacks in your car, desk, purse, and freezer, you'll never be left in the lurch.

FOR WHEN YOU...	HAVE THIS
Are running late in the morning and miss breakfast	**Kind Nuts & Spices in Madagascar Vanilla** *(210 cals.)*
Forget your lunch	**Amy's Light & Lean Spinach Lasagna** *(345 cals.)*
Need a 3 P.M. pick-me-up	**Blue Diamond Oven Roasted Almonds, Sea Salt** *(110-calorie pack)*
Have a late-night hankering	**Lifeway Tart and Tangy Pomegranate Frozen Kefir** *(90 calories per ½ cup)*

DAILY ASSESSMENT

● Did anything unexpected occur today? How did you cope? If you didn't cope well, how would you handle it in the future?

● Did you schedule in exercise and stick with it? If not, what changed your plans?

● Did you discover anything about food/movement/yourself today that you found helpful or motivating?

● What nice thing did you do for yourself today?

● Final thoughts on the day: Are you pleased with how the day went? What went well? What do you resolve to improve tomorrow?

✳ **DON'T FORGET** | *Check your to-do list before signing off for the night! It'll help you be ready for tomorrow.*

DAY 4

TO-DO LIST

- Assess your schedule for today. Is anything going to make it difficult to stick to your diet? Strategize to overcome obstacles.

- Put some formal exercise on today's calendar or think about extra ways you can move your body.

- Plan for tomorrow's meals tonight. What are you going to eat? Do you have everything you need? If you're brown-bagging tomorrow's lunch, save time by assembling what you can now.

- Pack your journal or make sure you have a pen and paper (or a smartphone) for making notes throughout the day.

- Remind yourself of the commitment you made—and of how great you're going to feel as you make progress.

STICK-TO-IT STRATEGY

See Yourself Younger and Thinner Chances are there was a time in your life when you felt more confident and carefree and looked younger, leaner, and healthier. Find a photo of yourself taken at that time and put it someplace prominent to remind yourself every day of how you were at your best. Seeing is believing—that you can be your old self again.

BREAKFAST

Hunger Level

FOOD/AMOUNT _____

_____

_____

_____

_____

_____

EMOTIONS _____

_____

_____

_____

_____

LUNCH

Hunger
Level

FOOD/AMOUNT _____

_____

_____

_____

_____

_____

_____

EMOTIONS _____

_____

_____

_____

_____

_____

DINNER

Hunger
Level

FOOD/AMOUNT _____

_____

_____

_____

_____

_____

_____

EMOTIONS _____

_____

_____

_____

_____

_____

SNACK 1

TIME/PLACE _____ *Hunger Level*

FOOD/AMOUNT _____

EMOTIONS _____

SNACK 2

TIME/PLACE _____ *Hunger Level*

FOOD/AMOUNT _____

EMOTIONS _____

UNPLANNED EATING

FOOD/AMOUNT _____ *Hunger Level*

TIME/PLACE _____

EMOTIONS _____

DAILY MOVEMENT

Type of Activity	Minutes/Amount	How It Felt
AEROBIC Exercises:		
STRENGTHENING Exercises:		
FLEXIBILITY Exercises:		
BALANCE Exercises:		
INCIDENTAL MOVEMENT		

Move More, Lose More

The Around-the-House Workout Time spent on chores is time well spent—in more ways than one. You'll burn 100 calories* when you devote:

- **20 minutes to weeding the garden**
- **25 minutes to vacuuming the rugs**
- **30 minutes to sweeping the floors**
- **35 minutes to dusting the house**
- **40 minutes to unloading the dryer and folding laundry**

Calories burned based on a 140-pound woman.

DAILY ASSESSMENT

- Did anything unexpected occur today? How did you cope? If you didn't cope well, how would you handle it in the future?

_____

_____

- Did you schedule in exercise and stick with it? If not, what changed your plans?

_____

_____

- Did you discover anything about food/movement/yourself today that you found helpful or motivating?

_____

_____

- What nice thing did you do for yourself today?

_____

_____

- Final thoughts on the day: Are you pleased with how the day went? What went well? What do you resolve to improve tomorrow?

_____

_____

_____

_____

_____

✻ DON'T FORGET | *Check your to-do list before signing off for the night! It'll help you be ready for tomorrow.*

TO-DO LIST

- Assess your schedule for today. Is anything going to make it difficult to stick to your diet? Strategize to overcome obstacles.

- Put some formal exercise on today's calendar or think about extra ways you can move your body.

- Plan for tomorrow's meals tonight. What are you going to eat? Do you have everything you need? If you're brown-bagging tomorrow's lunch, save time by assembling what you can now.

- Pack your journal or make sure you have a pen and paper (or a smartphone) for making notes throughout the day.

- Remind yourself of the commitment you made—and of how great you're going to feel as you make progress.

MORE MINDFUL EATING

Lay It On Thick Some foods may fill you up faster than others. Case in point: A British study found that people judged thick blended drinks to be more satisfying than thinner ones, regardless of calories. And that's a good thing: Just the prospect of a full belly can reduce your appetite and make you eat less. So thicken your smoothies with healthy nonfat Greek yogurt and frozen fruit.

BREAKFAST

Hunger Level

FOOD/AMOUNT _____

_____
_____
_____
_____

EMOTIONS _____

_____
_____
_____
_____
_____

LUNCH

Hunger Level

FOOD/AMOUNT _____

_____

_____

_____

_____

EMOTIONS _____

_____

_____

_____

_____

―――――――――――――――― TESTER TIP ――――――――――――――――

"If I have an 'off-the-wagon' moment, waking up
the next day to a simple 300-calorie breakfast
is the best way to get back on track. And I avoid
the scale until I've had more positive plan days."

—Porscha Burke, 7 pounds and 2 inches lost

DINNER

Hunger Level

FOOD/AMOUNT _____

_____

_____

_____

_____

EMOTIONS _____

_____

_____

_____

_____

SNACK 1

TIME/PLACE _____ *Hunger Level*

FOOD/AMOUNT _____

EMOTIONS _____

SNACK 2

TIME/PLACE _____ *Hunger Level*

FOOD/AMOUNT _____

EMOTIONS _____

UNPLANNED EATING

FOOD/AMOUNT _____ *Hunger Level*

TIME/PLACE _____

EMOTIONS _____

DAILY MOVEMENT

Type of Activity	Minutes/Amount	How It Felt
AEROBIC Exercises:		
STRENGTHENING Exercises:		
FLEXIBILITY Exercises:		
BALANCE Exercises:		
INCIDENTAL MOVEMENT		

Anti-Aging Eating

Healthy Vegetarian Choices Protein is a muscle booster and skin saver. And beans, nuts, and soy are great protein-packed alternatives to meat. Each option below has roughly the same calories as 3 ounces of cooked chicken breast (140).

PICK A PROTEIN	CALORIES
Fat-free refried beans *(2/3 cup)*	137
Almonds *(20 nuts)*	138
Kidney beans *(2/3 cup)*	139
Chickpeas *(2/3 cup)*	139
Peanut butter (smooth or chunky) *(1½ Tbsp.)*	141
Edamame *(¾ cup)*	143
Firm tofu *(6 oz.)*	143
Walnuts *(11 halves)*	144
Black beans *(2/3 cup)*	144
Peanuts *(25 nuts)*	146
Lentils *(2/3 cup cooked lentils)*	152

DAILY ASSESSMENT

● Did anything unexpected occur today? How did you cope? If you didn't cope well, how would you handle it in the future?

_____

● Did you schedule in exercise and stick with it? If not, what changed your plans?

_____

● Did you discover anything about food/movement/yourself today that you found helpful or motivating?

_____

● What nice thing did you do for yourself today?

_____

● Final thoughts on the day: Are you pleased with how the day went? What went well? What do you resolve to improve tomorrow?

_____

✳ DON'T FORGET	*Check your to-do list before signing off for the night! It'll help you be ready for tomorrow.*

DAY 6

TO-DO LIST

- Assess your schedule for today. Is anything going to make it difficult to stick to your diet? Strategize to overcome obstacles.

- Put some formal exercise on today's calendar or think about extra ways you can move your body.

- Plan for tomorrow's meals tonight. What are you going to eat? Do you have everything you need? If you're brown-bagging tomorrow's lunch, save time by assembling what you can now.

- Pack your journal or make sure you have a pen and paper (or a smartphone) for making notes throughout the day.

- Remind yourself of the commitment you made—and of how great you're going to feel as you make progress.

MOVE MORE, LOSE MORE

Cardio or Weights? You're strapped for time. So which do you do: a cardio workout or a weight-lifting workout? Research shows that cardio brings about more weight loss than resistance training. And don't feel bad if you can't do both: Study participants who did cardio and resistance training lost just a bit more than cardio-only exercisers—though they put in twice the time.

BREAKFAST

Hunger Level

FOOD/AMOUNT _____

_____

_____

_____

_____

_____

EMOTIONS _____

_____

_____

_____

_____

LUNCH

*Hunger
Level*

FOOD/AMOUNT _____

_____

_____

_____

_____

_____

_____

EMOTIONS _____

_____

_____

_____

_____

_____

DINNER

*Hunger
Level*

FOOD/AMOUNT _____

_____

_____

_____

_____

_____

_____

EMOTIONS _____

_____

_____

_____

_____

_____

SNACK 1

Hunger Level

TIME/PLACE _____

FOOD/AMOUNT _____

EMOTIONS _____

SNACK 2

Hunger Level

TIME/PLACE _____

FOOD/AMOUNT _____

EMOTIONS _____

UNPLANNED EATING

Hunger Level

FOOD/AMOUNT _____

TIME/PLACE _____

EMOTIONS _____

DAILY MOVEMENT

Type of Activity	Minutes/Amount	How It Felt
AEROBIC Exercises:		
STRENGTHENING Exercises:		
FLEXIBILITY Exercises:		
BALANCE Exercises:		
INCIDENTAL MOVEMENT		

Anti-Aging Eating

The Fiber Bonus A diet rich in fiber can not only help you lose weight, but also help you live a longer life. For every 7 grams of fiber you eat per day, you reduce your likelihood of stroke by 7%. Most Americans get only about 15 grams of fiber a day, not even close to the 25 grams the American Heart Association recommends. But since high-fiber foods—fruits, vegetables, whole grains, and beans—are pillars of the *7 Years Younger Anti-Aging Breakthrough Diet,* you can exceed that recommendation every day.

DAILY ASSESSMENT

● Did anything unexpected occur today? How did you cope? If you didn't cope well, how would you handle it in the future?

_____

_____

● Did you schedule in exercise and stick with it? If not, what changed your plans?

_____

_____

● Did you discover anything about food/movement/yourself today that you found helpful or motivating?

_____

_____

● What nice thing did you do for yourself today?

_____

_____

● Final thoughts on the day: Are you pleased with how the day went? What went well? What do you resolve to improve tomorrow?

_____

_____

_____

_____

_____

_____

| ✳ **DON'T FORGET** | *Check your to-do list before signing off for the night! It'll help you be ready for tomorrow.* |

TO-DO LIST

- Assess your schedule for today. Is anything going to make it difficult to stick to your diet? Strategize to overcome obstacles.

- Put some formal exercise on today's calendar or think about extra ways you can move your body.

- Plan for tomorrow's meals tonight. What are you going to eat? Do you have everything you need? If you're brown-bagging tomorrow's lunch, save time by assembling what you can now.

- Pack your journal or make sure you have a pen and paper (or a smartphone) for making notes throughout the day.

- Remind yourself of the commitment you made—and of how great you're going to feel as you make progress.

EMOTIONAL-EATING ALERT

People-Pleasing Calories Researchers at Case Western Reserve University invited volunteers to a meeting in which a staff member (actually an actor) passed around a bowl of M&M's. Those who scored higher on the sociotropy scale (a measure of one's need for social acceptance) took more than those less concerned about the comfort of others. Being nice is an excellent trait—but don't sacrifice your body to be sociable.

BREAKFAST

Hunger Level

FOOD/AMOUNT _____

_____

_____

_____

_____

EMOTIONS _____

_____

_____

LUNCH

Hunger Level

FOOD/AMOUNT _____

_____
_____
_____
_____
_____
_____
_____

EMOTIONS _____

_____
_____
_____
_____
_____

DINNER

Hunger Level

FOOD/AMOUNT _____

_____
_____
_____
_____
_____
_____
_____

EMOTIONS _____

_____
_____
_____
_____
_____

SNACK 1

Hunger Level

TIME/PLACE _____

FOOD/AMOUNT _____

EMOTIONS _____

SNACK 2

Hunger Level

TIME/PLACE _____

FOOD/AMOUNT _____

EMOTIONS _____

UNPLANNED EATING

Hunger Level

FOOD/AMOUNT _____

TIME/PLACE _____

EMOTIONS _____

DAILY MOVEMENT

Type of Activity	Minutes/Amount	How It Felt
AEROBIC Exercises:		
STRENGTHENING Exercises:		
FLEXIBILITY Exercises:		
BALANCE Exercises:		
INCIDENTAL MOVEMENT		

LUNCH

Weight-Loss Booster

Try these skinny substitutions and see how many calories you'll avoid consuming.

INSTEAD OF...	CHOOSE	CALORIES SAVED
5-ounce glass of wine	6-ounce wine spritzer	50
1 cup spaghetti	1 cup spaghetti squash	179
1/4 cup pancake syrup	1/2 cup frozen blueberries, microwaved	144
1 cup mashed potatoes	1 small baked sweet potato	183
2 slices Swiss cheese (on a sandwich)	1 serving Alouette Portions	173

DAILY ASSESSMENT

• Did anything unexpected occur today? How did you cope? If you didn't cope well, how would you handle it in the future?

_____

_____

• Did you schedule in exercise and stick with it? If not, what changed your plans?

_____

_____

• Did you discover anything about food/movement/yourself today that you found helpful or motivating?

_____

_____

• What nice thing did you do for yourself today?

_____

_____

• Final thoughts on the day: Are you pleased with how the day went? What went well? What do you resolve to improve tomorrow?

_____

_____

✳ **DON'T FORGET**	_Check your to-do list before signing off for the night! It'll help you be ready for tomorrow._

How Was Your Week?

By Week 4, it's not unusual to feel a little diet fatigue. That can lead to letting your guard down with sabotaging thoughts: "I've been so good, I deserve a bowl of ice cream"; "Going to the gym is just too hard, and I don't like exercising at home"; "It's rude not to join my friends in having nachos and margaritas." Have you had any similar self-defeating feelings or thoughts this week? Formulate some responses you can use to combat your negative thinking.

_____

_____

_____

_____

_____

_____

_____

_____

_____

_____

_____

GOALS FOR NEXT WEEK

_____

_____

_____

_____

_____

_____

_____

_____

_____

_____

WEEK 5

WEEK 5

DAY 1

Breakfast: Sunrise Soft Taco
Lunch: Finger Food
Snack 1: Honeydew "Sundae"
Dinner: Spice-Rubbed Pork Tenderloin
Snack 2: Cherries & Cheese

DAY 2

Breakfast: Breakfast to Go
Lunch: Garden Turkey Sandwich with Lemon Mayo
Snack 1: Strawberry Bagel Thin
Dinner: Healthy-Makeover Meatloaf
Snack 2: Cocoa Fix

DAY 3

Breakfast: Breakfast Pizza
Lunch: Mexican Meal in Minutes
Snack 1: Hummus & Veggie Strips
Dinner: Chicken with Berry Sauce
Snack 2: Prosciutto & Mozzarella Plate

DAY 4

Breakfast: New York Bagel
Lunch: Roast Beef Chef's Salad
Snack 1: PB & J–Inspired Yogurt
Dinner: Steamed Scrod Fillet Dinner
Snack 2: Out & About

DAY 5

Breakfast: Banana–Peanut Butter Smoothie
Lunch: Creole Chicken Frankfurter Meal
Snack 1: Chips & Cheese
Dinner: Curried Chicken Salad
Snack 2: Edamame Munchie

DAY 6

Breakfast: Easy Oatmeal
Lunch: Sandwich & Slaw
Snack 1: Citrus Snack
Dinner: Soba Noodle Bowl with Shrimp & Snow Peas
Snack 2: Movie Mix

DAY 7

Breakfast: Ham & Veggie Hash
Lunch: Easy Cobb Salad
Snack 1: Iced-Coffee Break
Dinner: Fajitas Two Ways
Snack 2: Pudding Parfait

Shopping List

For breakfasts, lunches, and dinners serving anywhere from one to six. Check recipes to make adjustments depending on the number of people you are feeding.

FRESH PRODUCE

- 1 teaspoon chives
- 1½ cups cilantro leaves
- 1 tablespoon mint leaves
- 1 tablespoon flat-leaf parsley leaves
- 4 green onions
- 1 small white or yellow onion
- 1 pint (12 ounces) grape or cherry tomatoes
- 1 plum tomato
- 2 regular tomatoes
- 1 pound bok choy
- 1 pound red cabbage
- 2 bags (5 to 6 ounces each) mixed salad greens
- 1 bag (10 ounces) romaine hearts
- 1 bag (5 to 6 ounces) baby spinach
- 3¼ cups shredded carrots
- 6 stalks celery
- 2 cups corn kernels (from about 4 ears)
- 1 seedless (English) cucumber
- 2 pounds green beans
- 5 mushrooms
- 1 large green bell pepper
- 1 medium and 1 large red bell pepper
- 6 medium red potatoes (1½ pounds total)
- 1 small sweet potato
- 4 ounces snow peas
- 1 small yellow summer squash
- 1 medium apple
- 2 bananas
- 1½ pints blackberries (18 ounces total)
- ¼ cup cantaloupe chunks
- 10 cherries
- 1 bag red grapes
- 1 pink grapefruit
- 1 honeydew melon
- 2 oranges
- 1 pear
- 3 large strawberries
- ¼ small watermelon

SEAFOOD

- 4 scrod fillets (1½ pounds total)
- 8 ounces (20- to 23-count) large raw shrimp, shelled and deveined
- 1 ounce lox

MEAT & POULTRY

- 8 ounces beef sirloin strip steak
- 1¼ pounds chicken-breast cutlets
- 2¼ pounds skinless, boneless chicken-breast halves
- 1 pound pork tenderloin
- 2 pounds lean ground turkey
- 6 slices fully cooked, ready-to-serve bacon
- 3 ounces lean roast beef
- 1 Applegate Farms Organic chicken hot dog
- 2 cups cooked chicken-breast meat
- 4 ounces thick-sliced ham or 4-ounce piece of ham
- ½ ounce very thinly sliced prosciutto
- 5 ounces thinly sliced low-sodium smoked turkey breast

DAIRY

- 1 Mini Babybel Light cheese
- 3 ounces blue cheese
- 1 wedge Laughing Cow ⅓ Less Fat Classic Cream Cheese Spread
- 3 tablespoons crumbled reduced-fat feta cheese

¾ ounce aged goat cheese or Brie

¼ cup shredded reduced-fat Monterey Jack cheese

1 ounce part-skim mozzarella cheese

1 stick part-skim mozzarella string cheese

½ cup low-fat (1%), low-sodium cottage cheese

1 container (4 ounces) Kozy Shack No-Sugar-Added Chocolate Pudding

1 container (6 ounces) sugar-free vanilla pudding

¼ cup reduced-fat sour cream

GRAIN PRODUCTS

1 cup whole wheat couscous

8 ounces 100% whole buckwheat soba noodles

1 whole-grain soft breadstick

1 whole wheat frankfurter bun

1 cup Uncle Ben's Ready Rice brown rice

FROZEN

7 Applegate Farms chicken nuggets

1½ cups frozen peas

MISCELLANEOUS

12 Emerald Cocoa Roast Almonds (dark-chocolate flavor)

1 Kind Mini Fruit & Nut Delight Bar

1 Kind Nuts & Spices Bar in Madagascar Vanilla Almond

1½ tablespoons bean dip

1 tea bag chai tea

⅓ cup prepared coleslaw

½ cup no-sugar-added frozen yogurt, flavor of your choice

¼ cup hummus

½ cup Edy's/Dreyer's Slow Churned No Sugar Added Ice Cream, vanilla flavor

1 cup Good Health Half Naked Popcorn

1 Healthy Choice Chicken Tortilla microwavable soup bowl

1 cup Imagine Creamy Portobello Mushroom Soup

22 SunChips

15 sweet potato chips

1 can (11½ ounces) low-sodium tomato or vegetable juice

5 Food Should Taste Good Multigrain tortilla chips

10 Triscuit Thin Crisps

TO-DO LIST

- Reread your pledge.

- Assess your schedule for today. Is anything going to make it difficult to stick to your diet? Strategize to overcome obstacles.

- Put some formal exercise on today's calendar or think about ways you can move your body.

- Plan for tomorrow's meals tonight. What are you going to eat? Do you have everything you need? If you're brown-bagging tomorrow's lunch, save time by assembling what you can now.

- Pack your journal or make sure you have a pen and paper (or a smartphone) for making notes throughout the day.

- Remind yourself of the commitment you made—and of how great you're going to feel as you make progress.

STICK-TO-IT STRATEGY

Scan the Horizon Each day, as you go over what you've written in this workbook, look back at how far you've come, not ahead at how much you have left to do. Scientists call this the "horizon effect" and note that it creates encouragement and builds determination. Reflecting on your accomplishments, big or small, will help provide ongoing inspiration.

BREAKFAST

Hunger Level

FOOD/AMOUNT _____

EMOTIONS _____

LUNCH

FOOD/AMOUNT _____

_____

_____

_____

_____

EMOTIONS _____

_____

_____

_____

_____

TESTER TIP

"I make two or three dinners on Sunday and alternate eating them throughout the week. That's enough for seven nights, so I don't default to my old habit of ordering in."

—Mary Marotta, 19 pounds and 7¾ inches lost

DINNER

Hunger
Level

FOOD/AMOUNT _____

_____

_____

_____

_____

EMOTIONS _____

_____

_____

_____

_____

SNACK 1

Hunger Level

TIME/PLACE _____

FOOD/AMOUNT _____

EMOTIONS _____

SNACK 2

Hunger Level

TIME/PLACE _____

FOOD/AMOUNT _____

EMOTIONS _____

UNPLANNED EATING

Hunger Level

FOOD/AMOUNT _____

TIME/PLACE _____

EMOTIONS _____

DAILY MOVEMENT

Type of Activity	Minutes/Amount	How It Felt
AEROBIC Exercises:		
STRENGTHENING Exercises:		
FLEXIBILITY Exercises:		
BALANCE Exercises:		
INCIDENTAL MOVEMENT		

Crazy-Busy-Proof Your Diet It's tough cooking during the week—and let's face it, there are nights when it's just not going to happen. But don't sweat it if you don't have time to fix dinner at night. Take a little time on the weekends to cook and freeze some great meals. You don't even have to do it every weekend, just about twice a month. As you go, precut and portion out everything so that instead of ordering in, you have a delicious "frozen" meal at the ready. It will be healthier than takeout and much tastier than anything your grocery store stocks.

DAILY ASSESSMENT

- Over these past few weeks, what has kept you going ("I can picture my new body at the end of seven weeks"; "I've never felt so energetic")? Turn whatever it is into a mantra you can repeat to yourself daily.

- Think about the people in your life. Did anyone help you stay on track today? Did anyone undermine you? Ponder how to get more healthy influences into your life—and eliminate or de-emphasize the negative ones.

- Did you schedule in exercise and stick with it? If not, what changed your plans?

- Did you discover anything about food/movement/yourself today that you found helpful or motivating?

- What nice thing did you do for yourself today?

- Final thoughts on the day: Are you pleased with how the day went? What went well? What do you resolve to change tomorrow?

| ✱ **DON'T FORGET** | *Check your to-do list before signing off for the night! It'll help you be ready for tomorrow.* |

DAY 2

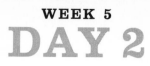

TO-DO LIST

- Assess your schedule for today. Is anything going to make it difficult to stick to your diet? Strategize to overcome obstacles.

- Put some formal exercise on today's calendar or think about extra ways you can move your body.

- Plan for tomorrow's meals tonight. What are you going to eat? Do you have everything you need? If you're brown-bagging tomorrow's lunch, save time by assembling what you can now.

- Pack your journal or make sure you have a pen and paper (or a smartphone) for making notes throughout the day.

- Remind yourself of the commitment you made—and of how great you're going to feel as you make progress.

WEIGHT-LOSS BOOSTER

Dressing Appropriately Sure, there are plenty of choices in the salad-dressing aisle, but which are healthiest? Look for ones that have about 45 calories per 2-tablespoon serving. Don't worry about fat—the fat in salad dressing tends to be of a healthy variety that helps boost nutrient absorption—but make sure the dressing has no more than 4 grams of sugar per serving. One good pick: Newman's Own Lite Balsamic.

BREAKFAST

Hunger Level

FOOD/AMOUNT _____

_____

_____

_____

_____

_____

EMOTIONS _____

_____

_____

_____

LUNCH

*Hunger
Level*

FOOD/AMOUNT _____

_____

_____

_____

_____

_____

_____

EMOTIONS _____

_____

_____

_____

_____

_____

DINNER

*Hunger
Level*

FOOD/AMOUNT _____

_____

_____

_____

_____

_____

_____

EMOTIONS _____

_____

_____

_____

_____

_____

SNACK 1

Hunger Level

TIME/PLACE _____

FOOD/AMOUNT _____

EMOTIONS _____

SNACK 2

Hunger Level

TIME/PLACE _____

FOOD/AMOUNT _____

EMOTIONS _____

UNPLANNED EATING

Hunger Level

FOOD/AMOUNT _____

TIME/PLACE _____

EMOTIONS _____

DAILY MOVEMENT

Type of Activity	Minutes/Amount	How It Felt
AEROBIC Exercises:		
STRENGTHENING Exercises:		
FLEXIBILITY Exercises:		
BALANCE Exercises:		
INCIDENTAL MOVEMENT		

Winning Winter Workouts Cold weather is the ultimate excuse for not getting in your usual walk, jog, or weekend hike. But these winter calorie-burners are just too effective to pass up. Consider...

Cross-country skiing	burns	630 calories/hour
Ice skating	burns	552 calories/hour
Downhill skiing	burns	474 calories/hour
Cold-weather walking	burns	300 calories/hour
Snowmobiling	burns	276 calories/hour
Bowling (for the cold-averse)	burns	237 calories/hour

DAILY ASSESSMENT

● Think about the people in your life. Did anyone help you stay on track today? Did anyone undermine you? Ponder how to get more healthy influences into your life— and eliminate or de-emphasize the negative ones.

● Did you schedule in exercise and stick with it? If not, what changed your plans?

● Did you discover anything about food/movement/yourself today that you found helpful or motivating?

● What nice thing did you do for yourself today?

● Final thoughts on the day: Are you pleased with how the day went? What went well? What do you resolve to improve tomorrow?

✷ **DON'T FORGET**	*Check your to-do list before signing off for the night! It'll help you be ready for tomorrow.*

TO-DO LIST

- Assess your schedule for today. Is anything going to make it difficult to stick to your diet? Strategize to overcome obstacles.

- Put some formal exercise on today's calendar or think about extra ways you can move your body.

- Plan for tomorrow's meals tonight. What are you going to eat? Do you have everything you need? If you're brown-bagging tomorrow's lunch, save time by assembling what you can now.

- Pack your journal or make sure you have a pen and paper (or a smartphone) for making notes throughout the day.

- Remind yourself of the commitment you made—and of how great you're going to feel as you make progress.

JUNK FOOD-JUNKIE ALERT

Help for Carboholics Switching to whole-grain carbs is healthier and can help you feel fuller on smaller portions. The best way to identify a good source of a whole grain? Look at the ratio of total carbs to fiber. A ratio of less than 10:1 (say, 24 grams of carbs to 3 grams of fiber, or 24÷3=8:1) indicates a good amount of whole grain but not too much sugar.

BREAKFAST

Hunger Level

FOOD/AMOUNT _____

_____

_____

_____

_____

EMOTIONS _____

_____

_____

_____

LUNCH

Hunger Level

FOOD/AMOUNT _____

_____

_____

_____

_____

_____

_____

_____

EMOTIONS _____

_____

_____

_____

_____

_____

DINNER

Hunger Level

FOOD/AMOUNT _____

_____

_____

_____

_____

_____

_____

_____

EMOTIONS _____

_____

_____

_____

_____

_____

SNACK 1

Hunger Level

TIME/PLACE _____

FOOD/AMOUNT _____

EMOTIONS _____

SNACK 2

Hunger Level

TIME/PLACE _____

FOOD/AMOUNT _____

EMOTIONS _____

UNPLANNED EATING

Hunger Level

FOOD/AMOUNT _____

TIME/PLACE _____

EMOTIONS _____

DAILY MOVEMENT

Type of Activity	Minutes/Amount	How It Felt
AEROBIC Exercises:		
STRENGTHENING Exercises:		
FLEXIBILITY Exercises:		
BALANCE Exercises:		
INCIDENTAL MOVEMENT		

Brain Food Milk, salmon, and tuna all have something in common: ample amounts of vitamin D, a nutrient that can help you stay sharp. In recent studies, older women with the highest blood levels of vitamin D had less cognitive decline, and those whose diets included lots of D-rich foods had a far lower risk of Alzheimer's. Other research has shown that, judging from the length of their telomeres (caps at the end of DNA strands that shorten with age), women with high levels of vitamin D are biologically *five years younger* than women with lower levels.

DAILY ASSESSMENT

- Think about the people in your life. Did anyone help you stay on track today? Did anyone undermine you? Ponder how to get more healthy influences into your life— and eliminate or de-emphasize the negative ones.

_____

_____

- Did you schedule in exercise and stick with it? If not, what changed your plans?

_____

_____

- Did you discover anything about food/movement/yourself today that you found helpful or motivating?

_____

_____

- What nice thing did you do for yourself today?

_____

_____

- Final thoughts on the day: Are you pleased with how the day went? What went well? What do you resolve to improve tomorrow?

_____

_____

_____

_____

_____

---

* DON'T FORGET | *Check your to-do list before signing off for the night! It'll help you be ready for tomorrow.*

DAY 4

TO-DO LIST

- Assess your schedule for today. Is anything going to make it difficult to stick to your diet? Strategize to overcome obstacles.

- Put some formal exercise on today's calendar or think about extra ways you can move your body.

- Plan for tomorrow's meals tonight. What are you going to eat? Do you have everything you need? If you're brown-bagging tomorrow's lunch, save time by assembling what you can now.

- Pack your journal or make sure you have a pen and paper (or a smartphone) for making notes throughout the day.

- Remind yourself of the commitment you made—and of how great you're going to feel as you make progress.

STICK-TO-IT STRATEGY

Always Exercise on Monday Starting the week with a walk or another type of physical activity can help you set the pace for the days that follow. It gets you off on the right foot by setting a psychological pattern, helping you make exercise a habit.

BREAKFAST

Hunger
Level

FOOD/AMOUNT _____

_____

_____

_____

_____

_____

EMOTIONS _____

_____

_____

_____

_____

LUNCH

Hunger Level

FOOD/AMOUNT _____

_____

_____

_____

_____

_____

_____

EMOTIONS _____

_____

_____

_____

_____

_____

DINNER

Hunger Level

FOOD/AMOUNT _____

_____

_____

_____

_____

_____

_____

EMOTIONS _____

_____

_____

_____

_____

_____

SNACK 1

Hunger Level

TIME/PLACE _____

FOOD/AMOUNT _____

EMOTIONS _____

SNACK 2

Hunger Level

TIME/PLACE _____

FOOD/AMOUNT _____

EMOTIONS _____

UNPLANNED EATING

Hunger Level

FOOD/AMOUNT _____

TIME/PLACE _____

EMOTIONS _____

DAILY MOVEMENT

Type of Activity	Minutes/Amount	How It Felt
AEROBIC Exercises:		
STRENGTHENING Exercises:		
FLEXIBILITY Exercises:		
BALANCE Exercises:		
INCIDENTAL MOVEMENT		

Make Your Middle Stronger It's short and sweet and guaranteed to help firm your abs: the plank. Lie facedown on the floor with your forearms resting beside your chest, your body forming a straight line. Curl your toes under and raise your body off the floor. It's similar to a push-up position, but with your forearms supporting the weight of your upper body. Pull your navel in toward your spine and hold for 10 to 20 seconds. Gradually extend the time you hold the position up to a minute (or more).

DAILY ASSESSMENT

- Think about the people in your life. Did anyone help you stay on track today? Did anyone undermine you? Ponder how to get more healthy influences into your life—and eliminate or de-emphasize the negative ones.

_____

_____

- Did you schedule in exercise and stick with it? If not, what changed your plans?

_____

_____

- Did you discover anything about food/movement/yourself today that you found helpful or motivating?

_____

_____

- What nice thing did you do for yourself today?

_____

- Final thoughts on the day: Are you pleased with how the day went? What went well? What do you resolve to improve tomorrow?

_____

_____

_____

_____

_____

_____

| ✳ **DON'T FORGET** | _Check your to-do list before signing off for the night!_ _It'll help you be ready for tomorrow._ |

TO-DO LIST

- Assess your schedule for today. Is anything going to make it difficult to stick to your diet? Strategize to overcome obstacles.

- Put some formal exercise on today's calendar or think about extra ways you can move your body.

- Plan for tomorrow's meals tonight. What are you going to eat? Do you have everything you need? If you're brown-bagging tomorrow's lunch, save time by assembling what you can now.

- Pack your journal or make sure you have a pen and paper (or a smartphone) for making notes throughout the day.

- Remind yourself of the commitment you made—and of how great you're going to feel as you make progress.

MORE MINDFUL EATING

Tweet the Pounds Away The more you tweet, the more pounds you may lose. That's what a University of North Carolina, Chapel Hill study found when looking at the Twitter habits of dieters. The microblogging site allows for accountability, provides support, and helps people stay focused on their goals, says study author Brie Turner-McGrievy, Ph.D.

BREAKFAST

Hunger Level

FOOD/AMOUNT _____

_____

_____

_____

_____

EMOTIONS _____

_____

_____

_____

_____

LUNCH

Hunger Level

FOOD/AMOUNT _____

_____

_____

_____

_____

EMOTIONS _____

_____

_____

_____

_____

=== TESTER TIP ===

"The next time you feel like cheating, get on the scale and chew a piece of gum instead."

—Eileen Cohen, 10½ pounds and 4½ inches lost

DINNER

Hunger Level

FOOD/AMOUNT _____

_____

_____

_____

_____

EMOTIONS _____

_____

_____

_____

_____

SNACK 1

Hunger Level

TIME/PLACE _____

FOOD/AMOUNT _____

EMOTIONS _____

SNACK 2

Hunger Level

TIME/PLACE _____

FOOD/AMOUNT _____

EMOTIONS _____

UNPLANNED EATING

Hunger Level

FOOD/AMOUNT _____

TIME/PLACE _____

EMOTIONS _____

DAILY MOVEMENT

Type of Activity	Minutes/Amount	How It Felt
AEROBIC Exercises:		
STRENGTHENING Exercises:		
FLEXIBILITY Exercises:		
BALANCE Exercises:		
INCIDENTAL MOVEMENT		

Read the Fine Print Over the past few years, more and more restaurants have begun posting nutritional information on menus and websites. That's good news; it can help you plan ahead and avoid being ambushed by extra calories. However, make sure that you check serving sizes as well as calorie counts so you don't end up eating two or more servings instead of just one. As a general rule, double up on veggies and lighten up on grains.

DAILY ASSESSMENT

- Think about the people in your life. Did anyone help you stay on track today? Did anyone undermine you? Ponder how to get more healthy influences into your life—and eliminate or de-emphasize the negative ones.

- Did you schedule in exercise and stick with it? If not, what changed your plans?

- Did you discover anything about food/movement/yourself today that you found helpful or motivating?

- What nice thing did you do for yourself today?

- Final thoughts on the day: Are you pleased with how the day went? What went well? What do you resolve to improve tomorrow?

| ✴ **DON'T FORGET** | *Check your to-do list before signing off for the night! It'll help you be ready for tomorrow.* |

TO-DO LIST

- Assess your schedule for today. Is anything going to make it difficult to stick to your diet? Strategize to overcome obstacles.

- Put some formal exercise on today's calendar or think about extra ways you can move your body.

- Plan for tomorrow's meals tonight. What are you going to eat? Do you have everything you need? If you're brown-bagging tomorrow's lunch, save time by assembling what you can now.

- Pack your journal or make sure you have a pen and paper (or a smartphone) for making notes throughout the day.

- Remind yourself of the commitment you made—and of how great you're going to feel as you make progress.

ANTI-AGING EATING

The Raw and the Cooked Devotees of the raw-food revolution argue that heating vegetables destroys the nutrients that help fight aging. But steaming or microwaving reduces vitamins only by about 15%. And some foods benefit from being cooked. Tomatoes' level of lycopene, a source of protection from sun damage and cancer, actually increases when the tomatoes are cooked.

BREAKFAST

Hunger Level

FOOD/AMOUNT _____

EMOTIONS _____

LUNCH

Hunger Level

FOOD/AMOUNT _____

_____

_____

_____

_____

_____

_____

EMOTIONS _____

_____

_____

_____

_____

DINNER

Hunger Level

FOOD/AMOUNT _____

_____

_____

_____

_____

_____

EMOTIONS _____

_____

_____

_____

_____

SNACK 1

TIME/PLACE _____

Hunger Level

FOOD/AMOUNT _____

EMOTIONS _____

SNACK 2

TIME/PLACE _____

Hunger Level

FOOD/AMOUNT _____

EMOTIONS _____

UNPLANNED EATING

FOOD/AMOUNT _____

Hunger Level

TIME/PLACE _____

EMOTIONS _____

DAILY MOVEMENT

Type of Activity	Minutes/Amount	How It Felt
AEROBIC Exercises:		
STRENGTHENING Exercises:		
FLEXIBILITY Exercises:		
BALANCE Exercises:		
INCIDENTAL MOVEMENT		

Got 10 Minutes? The next time you think you don't have enough time to exercise, reconsider. It takes just 10 minutes to **burn 101 calories**. Here's proof—with just four easy moves:

- **1 minute of lifting weights burns 7 calories**
- **3 minutes of jumping rope burns 36 calories**
- **3 minutes of jumping jacks burns 29 calories**
- **3 minutes of jogging in place burns 29 calories**

DAILY ASSESSMENT

- Think about the people in your life. Did anyone help you stay on track today? Did anyone undermine you? Ponder how to get more healthy influences into your life—and eliminate or de-emphasize the negative ones.

_____

_____

- Did you schedule in exercise and stick with it? If not, what changed your plans?

_____

- Did you discover anything about food/movement/yourself today that you found helpful or motivating?

_____

_____

- What nice thing did you do for yourself today?

_____

_____

- Final thoughts on the day: Are you pleased with how the day went? What went well? What do you resolve to improve tomorrow?

_____

_____

_____

_____

_____

* **DON'T FORGET** | *Check your to-do list before signing off for the night! It'll help you be ready for tomorrow.*

DAY 7

TO-DO LIST

- Assess your schedule for today. Is anything going to make it difficult to stick to your diet? Strategize to overcome obstacles.

- Put some formal exercise on today's calendar or think about extra ways you can move your body.

- Plan for tomorrow's meals tonight. What are you going to eat? Do you have everything you need? If you're brown-bagging tomorrow's lunch, save time by assembling what you can now.

- Pack your journal or make sure you have a pen and paper (or a smartphone) for making notes throughout the day.

- Remind yourself of the commitment you made—and of how great you're going to feel as you make progress.

WEIGHT-LOSS BOOSTER

50-Calorie Savory Snacks You can swap two of these for one savory meal-plan snack. Just be sure to pick produce whenever possible to make sure you get its anti-aging nutrients. **1.** 1 Ak-Mak Stone Ground Whole Wheat Sesame Cracker with 1 Tbsp. mashed avocado **2.** 1½ tablespoons hummus with ½ small red pepper, sliced for dipping **3.** 1 tablespoon soft herbed goat cheese with 1 stalk celery **4.** 10 baby carrots with 2 tablespoons salsa for dipping

BREAKFAST

Hunger Level

FOOD/AMOUNT _____

_____

_____

_____

_____

_____

EMOTIONS _____

_____

_____

_____

LUNCH

Hunger Level

FOOD/AMOUNT _____

_____

_____

_____

_____

_____

_____

_____

EMOTIONS _____

_____

_____

_____

_____

_____

DINNER

Hunger Level

FOOD/AMOUNT _____

_____

_____

_____

_____

_____

_____

EMOTIONS _____

_____

_____

_____

_____

_____

SNACK 1

Hunger Level

TIME/PLACE _____

FOOD/AMOUNT _____

EMOTIONS _____

SNACK 2

Hunger Level

TIME/PLACE _____

FOOD/AMOUNT _____

EMOTIONS _____

UNPLANNED EATING

Hunger Level

FOOD/AMOUNT _____

TIME/PLACE _____

EMOTIONS _____

DAILY MOVEMENT

Type of Activity	Minutes/Amount	How It Felt
AEROBIC Exercises:		
STRENGTHENING Exercises:		
FLEXIBILITY Exercises:		
BALANCE Exercises:		
INCIDENTAL MOVEMENT		

Fast-Food Cheat Sheet If getting three meals into your day means a stop at a fast-food restaurant, so be it. Just be sure to use the lower-calorie ordering lingo at your favorite chain to ensure that you won't exceed your day's calorie limits. To know before you go:

- **At Popeyes:** Order "blackened" chicken (from the Louisiana Live Well menu), which isn't battered or breaded *(320 fewer calories in a Chicken Po' Boy)*
- **At In-N-Out Burger:** Order a "protein-style" burger, which is wrapped in lettuce instead of a bun *(150 fewer calories in a regular hamburger)*
- **At Bruegger's:** Order a "skinny" bagel, which has the inner third removed *(100 fewer calories in a bagel or bagel sandwich)*
- **At Starbucks:** Order a "short" latte—an option that isn't on the menu but will get you an 8-ounce drink *(50 fewer calories than a tall latte)*
- **At Taco Bell:** Order a "fresco-style" meal, which swaps fresh Pico de Gallo for cheese- and dairy-based sauces *(50 fewer calories in a Steak Burrito Supreme)*

DAILY ASSESSMENT

- Think about the people in your life. Did anyone help you stay on track today? Did anyone undermine you? Ponder how to get more healthy influences into your life— and eliminate or de-emphasize the negative ones.

- Did you schedule in exercise and stick with it? If not, what changed your plans?

- Did you discover anything about food/movement/yourself today that you found helpful or motivating?

- What nice thing did you do for yourself today?

- Final thoughts on the day: Are you pleased with how the day went? What went well? What do you resolve to improve tomorrow?

✳ DON'T FORGET | *Check your to-do list before signing off for the night! It'll help you be ready for tomorrow.*

How Was Your Week?

A top goal of the 7 *Years Younger Anti-Aging Breakthrough Diet* is helping you to develop healthy new habits. Think back over your week and name five (or more) new habits you've adopted. Some examples: "I've stopped reading while eating lunch so that I can pay better attention to how full I am"; "I set my alarm a half hour earlier and take a walk in the morning"; "I brew a pot of chamomile tea in the evening to keep myself from snacking." What other habits are you still striving to adopt? Consider how you can make them a part of your life.

_____

_____

_____

_____

_____

_____

_____

_____

_____

_____

_____

GOALS FOR NEXT WEEK

_____

_____

_____

_____

_____

_____

_____

_____

_____

WEEK 6

WEEK 6

DAY 1

Breakfast: Sweet Stuffed Waffle
Lunch: Peanut Butter & Apple Sandwich
Snack 1: Pistachios
Dinner: Chipotle-Orange–Glazed Salmon
Snack 2: Cheese Bite

DAY 2

Breakfast: New York Bagel
Lunch: Spinach & Nectarine Salad
Snack 1: Iced-Coffee Break
Dinner: Steak & Oven Fries
Snack 2: Fruit & Grain Bar

DAY 3

Breakfast: Breakfast to Go
Lunch: Veggie Burger
Snack 1: Cantaloupe Boat
Dinner: Lemon-Oregano Chicken Cutlets
with Mint Zucchini
Snack 2: Strawberry Sipper

DAY 4

Breakfast: Huevos Rancheros
Lunch: Tuna & Cannellini Bean Salad
Snack 1: Cherries & Cheese
Dinner: Turkey-Escarole Soup
Snack 2: Veggies & Dill Dip

DAY 5

Breakfast: Berry Blast Breakfast Shake
Lunch: Creole Chicken Frankfurter Meal
Snack 1: Ricotta-Fig Toasts
Dinner: Big Fusilli Bowl
Snack 2: Prosciutto & Mozzarella Plate

DAY 6

Breakfast: 5-Minute Multigrain Cereal
Lunch: Subway Sandwich & Soup
Snack 1: Citrus Snack
Dinner: Scallop &
Cherry Tomato Skewers
Snack 2: Out & About

DAY 7

Breakfast: Grab & Go
Lunch: No-Cook Bean Burrito
Snack 1: Cocoa Fix
Dinner: Chicken Parm Stacks
Snack 2: Yogurt Sundae

Shopping List

For breakfasts, lunches, and dinners serving anywhere from one to six. Check recipes to make adjustments depending on the number of people you are feeding.

FRESH PRODUCE

- 3 tablespoons basil leaves
- ¾ cup cilantro leaves
- 1 teaspoon dill
- ⅔ cup mint leaves
- 1 tablespoon oregano leaves
- ½ cup flat-leaf parsley leaves
- 2 green onions
- 3 pints (12 ounces each) grape or cherry tomatoes
- 5 medium regular tomatoes
- 2 heads escarole
- 2 bags (5 to 6 ounces each) mixed greens or baby arugula
- 2 bags (9 ounces each) microwave-in-the-bag spinach
- 1 pound broccoli florets
- 2 cups shredded carrots
- 1 cup corn kernels (from about 2 ears)
- 1 small red bell pepper
- 3 baking potatoes (1½ pounds total)
- 1 small sweet potato
- 1 bunch radishes
- 1 pound yellow summer squash
- 4 medium zucchini
- 2 avocados
- 2 medium apples
- 1 half-pint (6 ounces) blackberries or blueberries
- 1 small cantaloupe
- 30 cherries
- 5 grapes
- 1 pink grapefruit
- 1 honeydew melon
- 2 nectarines
- 1 orange
- 1 plum
- 5 raspberries
- ¼ small watermelon

SEAFOOD

- 4 pieces skinless salmon fillet (1¼ pounds total)
- 16 large sea scallops
- 1 ounce lox
- 12 ounces light tuna packed in water

MEAT & POULTRY

- 1¼ pounds beef flank steak
- 1 pound chicken-breast cutlets
- 4 medium skinless, boneless chicken-breast halves (1½ pounds total)
- 1 Applegate Farms Organic chicken hot dog
- ½ ounce very thinly sliced prosciutto
- 2 cups chopped rotisserie chicken-breast meat

DAIRY

- 1 Mini Babybel Sharp Original or Gouda cheese
- 1 slice reduced-fat sharp Cheddar cheese
- 1 tablespoon Philadelphia ⅓ Less Fat Chive & Onion Cream Cheese
- ¾ ounce aged goat cheese or Brie
- 3 ounces part-skim mozzarella cheese
- 1 container (3½ ounces) Chobani Bites Raspberry with Dark Chocolate Chips

1 cup low-fat (1%), low-sodium
cottage cheese

3 tablespoons tzatziki sauce

GRAIN PRODUCTS

12 ounces whole-grain
fusilli pasta

½ cup whole wheat orzo pasta

2 ounces whole-grain spaghetti

2 tablespoons quick-cooking barley

1 whole wheat frankfurter bun

1 cup quinoa

FROZEN

2 Van's 8 Whole Grains waffles

1 black bean veggie burger

1¾ cups frozen sliced strawberries
or berry medley

CANNED GOODS

1 can (15 ounces) black beans

½ cup refried beans

2 cans (15 ounces each) white kidney
(cannellini) beans

3 cans (14½ ounces each)
low-sodium chicken broth

1 chipotle chile in adobo sauce

¼ cup marinara sauce

1 can (28 ounces) whole peeled
tomatoes in juice

MISCELLANEOUS

12 Emerald Cocoa Roast Almonds
(dark-chocolate flavor)

1 Kashi Chewy Cherry Dark
Chocolate Granola Bar

1 Kind Mini Fruit & Nut
Delight Bar

1 Kind Nuts & Spices Bar in
Madagascar Vanilla Almond

2 tablespoons Wholly Guacamole
All Natural Classic Guacamole

1 jar (4 ounces) sliced
pimientos

12 whole-grain pita chips

1 can (11½ ounces) low-sodium
tomato or vegetable juice

10 Multigrain Wheat Thins

8 (8-inch) bamboo skewers

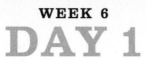

TO-DO LIST

- Reread your pledge.

- Assess your schedule for today. Is anything going to make it difficult to stick to your diet? Strategize to overcome obstacles.

- Put some formal exercise on today's calendar or think about ways you can move your body.

- Plan for tomorrow's meals tonight. What are you going to eat? Do you have everything you need? If you're brown-bagging tomorrow's lunch, save time by assembling what you can now.

- Pack your journal or make sure you have a pen and paper (or a smartphone) for making notes throughout the day.

- Remind yourself of the commitment you made—and of how great you're going to feel as you make progress.

LIQUID-CALORIE-LOVER ALERT

Coffee Considerations These "coffee drinks" can come at a high calorie cost. They should make you rethink your order (iced skim latte, anyone?):

Starbucks Venti Caffè Vanilla Frappuccino Blended Coffee with Whipped Cream—*530 calories*

Dunkin' Donuts large Frozen Coffee Coolatta with Cream—*860 calories*

McDonald's large McCafé Mocha with Whole Milk—*500 calories*

BREAKFAST

Hunger Level

FOOD/AMOUNT _____

_____

_____

_____

_____

EMOTIONS _____

_____

_____

_____

LUNCH

Hunger
Level

FOOD/AMOUNT _____

_____

_____

_____

_____

EMOTIONS _____

_____

_____

_____

_____

=============== TESTER TIP ===============

"With my homemade chicken stock I make a
soup filled with veggies, and I eat a bowl
when I get hungry. It's a freebie as long as
there are no added oils."

—*Debbie Hoch Barnard, 12¾ pounds and 3 inches lost*

DINNER

Hunger
Level

FOOD/AMOUNT _____

_____

_____

_____

_____

EMOTIONS _____

_____

_____

_____

_____

SNACK 1

Hunger Level

TIME/PLACE _____

FOOD/AMOUNT _____

EMOTIONS _____

SNACK 2

Hunger Level

TIME/PLACE _____

FOOD/AMOUNT _____

EMOTIONS _____

UNPLANNED EATING

Hunger Level

FOOD/AMOUNT _____

TIME/PLACE _____

EMOTIONS _____

DAILY MOVEMENT

Type of Activity	Minutes/Amount	How It Felt
AEROBIC Exercises:		
STRENGTHENING Exercises:		
FLEXIBILITY Exercises:		
BALANCE Exercises:		
INCIDENTAL MOVEMENT		

Stick-To-It Strategy

How to Address a Plateau Those points where weight loss slows or even stops temporarily are bound to come. But consider: Losing ½ pound a week is still losing, and that means you're still on track. If the scale isn't budging, read through your journal. Could some old habits be creeping back? Try returning to the Jumpstart week, which will likely nudge your body back into losing mode. Or, experiment with a new form of exercise. "Our bodies adapt to the same old thing," says GHRI Nutrition Director Sam Cassetty, "so if you're used to walking, you may want to try cycling, or even interval walking—bumping up the pace for a minute until you're really out of breath and then easing off for a few minutes."

DAILY ASSESSMENT

- Losing weight and adhering to a meal plan can bring about changes that extend beyond the number displayed on your scale. Now that you're in Week 6, are there other aspects of your life that feel different? What can you do to maintain those positive changes?

- What was your stress level today? If it was high, is there something you can do to alleviate it for tomorrow?

- Did you schedule in exercise and follow through? If not, what changed your plans?

- Did you discover anything about food/movement/yourself today that you found helpful or motivating?

- What nice thing did you do for yourself today?

- Final thoughts on the day: Are you pleased with how the day went? What went well? What do you resolve to change tomorrow?

✽ **DON'T FORGET** | *Check your to-do list before signing off for the night! It'll help you be ready for tomorrow.*

DAY 2

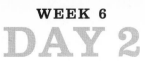

TO-DO LIST

- Assess your schedule for today. Is anything going to make it difficult to stick to your diet? Strategize to overcome obstacles.

- Put some formal exercise on today's calendar or think about extra ways you can move your body.

- Plan for tomorrow's meals tonight. What are you going to eat? Do you have everything you need? If you're brown-bagging tomorrow's lunch, save time by assembling what you can now.

- Pack your journal or make sure you have a pen and paper (or a smartphone) for making notes throughout the day.

- Remind yourself of the commitment you made—and of how great you're going to feel as you make progress.

MOVE MORE, LOSE MORE

The Mind-Body Burn Workouts that have a meditative or mind-focusing component are beloved for their stress-reducing and flexibility- and strength-building benefits, but usually are not thought of as calorie-burners. Yet in fact, a mind-body session does work off a nice chunk of calories. Here are the stats (per half hour) for a 140-pound woman:

Power yoga = *223*   **Pilates =** *117*   **Tai chi =** *133*   **Ballet =** *133*

BREAKFAST

Hunger Level

FOOD/AMOUNT _____

_____

_____

_____

_____

_____

EMOTIONS _____

_____

_____

_____

_____

LUNCH

Hunger Level

FOOD/AMOUNT _____

_____

_____

_____

_____

_____

_____

EMOTIONS _____

_____

_____

_____

_____

_____

DINNER

Hunger Level

FOOD/AMOUNT _____

_____

_____

_____

_____

_____

_____

EMOTIONS _____

_____

_____

_____

_____

_____

SNACK 1

Hunger Level

TIME/PLACE _____

FOOD/AMOUNT _____

EMOTIONS _____

SNACK 2

Hunger Level

TIME/PLACE _____

FOOD/AMOUNT _____

EMOTIONS _____

UNPLANNED EATING

Hunger Level

FOOD/AMOUNT _____

TIME/PLACE _____

EMOTIONS _____

DAILY MOVEMENT

Type of Activity	Minutes/Amount	How It Felt
AEROBIC Exercises:		
STRENGTHENING Exercises:		
FLEXIBILITY Exercises:		
BALANCE Exercises:		
INCIDENTAL MOVEMENT		

Snackalicious! Expand your snack horizons. These hunger-stoppers (each 120 calories or less) will slide just as easily into your bag as they do into your kids' lunch boxes.

- **Mann's Snacks on the Go! Celery, Carrots & Grape Tomatoes With Ranch Dip Tray** *(80 calories)*
- **Sargento Natural Blends Double Cheddar Cheese Snacks** *(90 calories)*
- **Frito-Lay SunChips Harvest Cheddar Snacks** *(100 calories)*
- **Earth's Best Sweet Potato Cinnamon Pop Snax** *(60 calories)*
- **Chobani Champions Vanilla Chocolate Chunk Greek Yogurt** *(120 calories)*

DAILY ASSESSMENT

- What was your stress level today? If it was high, is there something you can do to alleviate it for tomorrow?

_____

_____

- Did you schedule in exercise and follow through? If not, what changed your plans?

_____

_____

- Did you discover anything about food/movement/yourself today that you found helpful or motivating?

_____

_____

- What nice thing did you do for yourself today?

_____

_____

- Final thoughts on the day: Are you pleased with how the day went? What went well? What do you resolve to change tomorrow?

_____

_____

_____

_____

✴ DON'T FORGET | *Check your to-do list before signing off for the night! It'll help you be ready for tomorrow.*

TO-DO LIST

- Assess your schedule for today. Is anything going to make it difficult to stick to your diet? Strategize to overcome obstacles.

- Put some formal exercise on today's calendar or think about extra ways you can move your body.

- Plan for tomorrow's meals tonight. What are you going to eat? Do you have everything you need? If you're brown-bagging tomorrow's lunch, save time by assembling what you can now.

- Pack your journal or make sure you have a pen and paper (or a smartphone) for making notes throughout the day.

- Remind yourself of the commitment you made—and of how great you're going to feel as you make progress.

ANTI-AGING EATING

Eggs: Back on the Grocery List If you haven't heard the news, let us be the first to tell you: Most people can eat an egg every day without fear of heart attack or stroke. A review of eight studies looking at the effects of egg-eating found that despite the cholesterol in their yolks, eggs are a healthy source of fill-you-up protein.

BREAKFAST

Hunger Level

FOOD/AMOUNT _____

_____

_____

_____

_____

EMOTIONS _____

_____

_____

_____

LUNCH

Hunger Level

FOOD/AMOUNT _____

_____

_____

_____

_____

_____

_____

EMOTIONS _____

_____

_____

_____

_____

_____

DINNER

Hunger Level

FOOD/AMOUNT _____

_____

_____

_____

_____

_____

_____

EMOTIONS _____

_____

_____

_____

_____

SNACK 1

Hunger
Level

TIME/PLACE _____

FOOD/AMOUNT _____

EMOTIONS _____

SNACK 2

Hunger
Level

TIME/PLACE _____

FOOD/AMOUNT _____

EMOTIONS _____

UNPLANNED EATING

Hunger
Level

FOOD/AMOUNT _____

TIME/PLACE _____

EMOTIONS _____

DAILY MOVEMENT

Type of Activity	Minutes/Amount	How It Felt
AEROBIC Exercises:		
STRENGTHENING Exercises:		
FLEXIBILITY Exercises:		
BALANCE Exercises:		
INCIDENTAL MOVEMENT		

Emotional-Eater Alert

Fatigue's Double Whammy Not only does sleepiness exacerbate the stress, anxiety, and sadness that lead to overeating, but it can also make you more likely to succumb to the temptation of cookies and cake. Researchers at McLean Hospital in Belmont, MA, showed people pictures of high-calorie goodies, then looked at their brains with functional-MRI machines. Those who had earlier reported daytime sleepiness had lower activity in the willpower-regulating areas of their brains than when they viewed photos of fruit and salads. Moral of the story: Get a good night's sleep (or sneak in a nap) to help you control your calorie intake.

DAILY ASSESSMENT

○ What was your stress level today? If it was high, is there something you can do to alleviate it for tomorrow?

_____

_____

○ Did you schedule in exercise and follow through? If not, what changed your plans?

_____

_____

○ Did you discover anything about food/movement/yourself today that you found helpful or motivating?

_____

_____

○ What nice thing did you do for yourself today?

_____

_____

○ Final thoughts on the day: Are you pleased with how the day went? What went well? What do you resolve to change tomorrow?

_____

_____

_____

_____

✱ DON'T FORGET | *Check your to-do list before signing off for the night! It'll help you be ready for tomorrow.*

TO-DO LIST

- Assess your schedule for today. Is anything going to make it difficult to stick to your diet? Strategize to overcome obstacles.

- Put some formal exercise on today's calendar or think about extra ways you can move your body.

- Plan for tomorrow's meals tonight. What are you going to eat? Do you have everything you need? If you're brown-bagging tomorrow's lunch, save time by assembling what you can now.

- Pack your journal or make sure you have a pen and paper (or a smartphone) for making notes throughout the day.

- Remind yourself of the commitment you made—and of how great you're going to feel as you make progress.

WEIGHT-LOSS BOOSTER

Water Works When you're exercising, nothing can make you feel fatigued faster than dehydration. And once you start craving water, you're already 3% dehydrated. To avoid becoming parched (especially in hot weather), drink two to three cups a few hours before you work out. Then, 10 minutes beforehand, have another cup. Then sip as you go, about one cup of water every 15 to 20 minutes.

BREAKFAST

Hunger Level

FOOD/AMOUNT _____

_____

_____

_____

_____

_____

EMOTIONS _____

_____

_____

_____

_____

LUNCH

*Hunger
Level*

FOOD/AMOUNT _____

_____
_____
_____
_____
_____
_____
_____

EMOTIONS _____

_____
_____
_____
_____
_____

DINNER

*Hunger
Level*

FOOD/AMOUNT _____

_____
_____
_____
_____
_____
_____

EMOTIONS _____

_____
_____
_____
_____
_____

SNACK 1

Hunger Level

TIME/PLACE _____

FOOD/AMOUNT _____

EMOTIONS _____

SNACK 2

Hunger Level

TIME/PLACE _____

FOOD/AMOUNT _____

EMOTIONS _____

UNPLANNED EATING

Hunger Level

FOOD/AMOUNT _____

TIME/PLACE _____

EMOTIONS _____

DAILY MOVEMENT

Type of Activity	Minutes/Amount	How It Felt
AEROBIC Exercises:		
STRENGTHENING Exercises:		
FLEXIBILITY Exercises:		
BALANCE Exercises:		
INCIDENTAL MOVEMENT		

Stick-To-It Strategy

Motivation Tips From the Trenches

How do GH readers stay motivated to exercise?

"I lost weight by exercising daily along with reducing fat, sugar, and portions and eating more fruit and veggies. I stuck to it because after I dropped 10 pounds, I got to go shopping!"
—*Claudia Birney, GH Facebook friend*

"Knowing that my friend is waiting to walk with me has gotten me going for 16 years!"
—*Anne Siegrist, GH Facebook friend*

DAILY ASSESSMENT

- What was your stress level today? If it was high, is there something you can do to alleviate it for tomorrow?

_____

_____

- Did you schedule in exercise and follow through? If not, what changed your plans?

_____

_____

- Did you discover anything about food/movement/yourself today that you found helpful or motivating?

_____

_____

- What nice thing did you do for yourself today?

_____

_____

- Final thoughts on the day: Are you pleased with how the day went? What went well? What do you resolve to change tomorrow?

_____

_____

_____

✻ DON'T FORGET | *Check your to-do list before signing off for the night! It'll help you be ready for tomorrow.*

TO-DO LIST

- Assess your schedule for today. Is anything going to make it difficult to stick to your diet? Strategize to overcome obstacles.

- Put some formal exercise on today's calendar or think about extra ways you can move your body.

- Plan for tomorrow's meals tonight. What are you going to eat? Do you have everything you need? If you're brown-bagging tomorrow's lunch, save time by assembling what you can now.

- Pack your journal or make sure you have a pen and paper (or a smartphone) for making notes throughout the day.

- Remind yourself of the commitment you made—and of how great you're going to feel as you make progress.

MINDLESS-MUNCHER ALERT

Best Dining-Out Advice If you happen to be at a spot that lists calories on the menu, remember the *7 Years Younger Anti-Aging Breakthrough Diet* simple rule of 3, 4, 5—around 300 calories for breakfast, 400 for lunch, and 500 for dinner. No calorie information? Fill up on produce-rich meals—salad with a lean protein (like grilled chicken or shrimp) is a perfect example. Be careful with grain foods like pasta and rice: Restaurant portions can be over the top.

BREAKFAST

Hunger Level

FOOD/AMOUNT _____

_____
_____
_____
_____

EMOTIONS _____

_____
_____
_____
_____
_____

LUNCH

FOOD/AMOUNT _____

Hunger Level

EMOTIONS _____

TESTER TIP

"I went to a black-tie gala and had four club sodas with lime, six shrimp, four pieces of celery, and four pieces of red pepper. I was so proud, and my husband loved having a driver."

—*Jeanne Fishwick, 8 pounds, 2¾ inches lost*

DINNER

FOOD/AMOUNT _____

Hunger Level

EMOTIONS _____

SNACK 1

Hunger Level

TIME/PLACE _____

FOOD/AMOUNT _____

EMOTIONS _____

SNACK 2

Hunger Level

TIME/PLACE _____

FOOD/AMOUNT _____

EMOTIONS _____

UNPLANNED EATING

Hunger Level

FOOD/AMOUNT _____

TIME/PLACE _____

EMOTIONS _____

DAILY MOVEMENT

Type of Activity	Minutes/Amount	How It Felt
AEROBIC Exercises:		
STRENGTHENING Exercises:		
FLEXIBILITY Exercises:		
BALANCE Exercises:		
INCIDENTAL MOVEMENT		

Stick-To-It Strategy

Compare and Contrast You wind up in a fast-food restaurant. How to navigate? Look for the best option, of course! Here, we've done the math so you can see how to play it smart. Have *one* from the right-hand column and save mega calories!

1 Taco Bell XXL Grilled Stuft Steak Burrito *(850 calories)*	=	3 Taco Bell Steak Gordita Supremes *(280 calories each)*
1 Johnny Rockets Bacon Cheddar Double *(1,770 calories)*	=	3.5 Johnny Rockets Bacon, Lettuce, & Tomato Sandwiches *(480 calories each)*
1 Baja Fresh Chicken Tostada salad *(1,140 calories)*	=	3 Chicken Baja Ensalada salads with fat-free salsa verde *(325 calories each)*

DAILY ASSESSMENT

● What was your stress level today? If it was high, is there something you can do to alleviate it for tomorrow?

_____

_____

● Did you schedule in exercise and follow through? If not, what changed your plans?

_____

_____

● Did you discover anything about food/movement/yourself today that you found helpful or motivating?

_____

_____

● What nice thing did you do for yourself today?

_____

_____

● Final thoughts on the day: Are you pleased with how the day went? What went well? What do you resolve to change tomorrow?

_____

_____

✳ DON'T FORGET | *Check your to-do list before signing off for the night! It'll help you be ready for tomorrow.*

TO-DO LIST

- Assess your schedule for today. Is anything going to make it difficult to stick to your diet? Strategize to overcome obstacles.

- Put some formal exercise on today's calendar or think about extra ways you can move your body.

- Plan for tomorrow's meals tonight. What are you going to eat? Do you have everything you need? If you're brown-bagging tomorrow's lunch, save time by assembling what you can now.

- Pack your journal or make sure you have a pen and paper (or a smartphone) for making notes throughout the day.

- Remind yourself of the commitment you made—and of how great you're going to feel as you make progress.

ANTI-AGING EATING

Say "Nuts" to Wrinkles! Vitamin E has moisturizing and anti-inflammatory properties that have been shown to help diminish the effects of sun damage and inhibit the processes that cause skin aging. Some of your best sources: nuts, nut butters, seeds, and oils made from seeds like canola.

BREAKFAST

Hunger Level

FOOD/AMOUNT _____

_____

_____

_____

_____

_____

EMOTIONS _____

_____

_____

_____

LUNCH

Hunger
Level

FOOD/AMOUNT _____

_____

_____

_____

_____

_____

_____

_____

EMOTIONS _____

_____

_____

_____

_____

_____

DINNER

Hunger
Level

FOOD/AMOUNT _____

_____

_____

_____

_____

_____

_____

EMOTIONS _____

_____

_____

_____

_____

_____

SNACK 1

Hunger Level

TIME/PLACE _____

FOOD/AMOUNT _____

EMOTIONS _____

SNACK 2

Hunger Level

TIME/PLACE _____

FOOD/AMOUNT _____

EMOTIONS _____

UNPLANNED EATING

Hunger Level

FOOD/AMOUNT _____

TIME/PLACE _____

EMOTIONS _____

DAILY MOVEMENT

Type of Activity	Minutes/Amount	How It Felt
AEROBIC Exercises:		
STRENGTHENING Exercises:		
FLEXIBILITY Exercises:		
BALANCE Exercises:		
INCIDENTAL MOVEMENT		

Move More, Lose More

Stand Up for Yourself Sitting does your health and weight no favors, so what to do if you're stuck with a sedentary job? It turns out that just getting up from your chair as often as possible lowers your risk of age-accelerating inflammation and heart disease and trims your waistline (compared with people who hardly get up at all). Says Genevieve Healy, Ph.D., author of an Australian study that looked at the difference between sitting and standing, "Stand up at least every 30 minutes." Even a brief pop-up helps.

DAILY ASSESSMENT

● What was your stress level today? If it was high, is there something you can do to alleviate it for tomorrow?

_____

_____

● Did you schedule in exercise and follow through? If not, what changed your plans?

_____

_____

● Did you discover anything about food/movement/yourself today that you found helpful or motivating?

_____

_____

● What nice thing did you do for yourself today?

_____

_____

● Final thoughts on the day: Are you pleased with how the day went? What went well? What do you resolve to change tomorrow?

_____

_____

_____

_____

_____

_____

| **✳ DON'T FORGET** | _Check your to-do list before signing off for the night! It'll help you be ready for tomorrow._ |

TO-DO LIST

- Assess your schedule for today. Is anything going to make it difficult to stick to your diet? Strategize to overcome obstacles.

- Put some formal exercise on today's calendar or think about extra ways you can move your body.

- Plan for tomorrow's meals tonight. What are you going to eat? Do you have everything you need? If you're brown-bagging tomorrow's lunch, save time by assembling what you can now.

- Pack your journal or make sure you have a pen and paper (or a smartphone) for making notes throughout the day.

- Remind yourself of the commitment you made—and of how great you're going to feel as you make progress.

CRAVINGS CONTROL

A Hint of Mint Consider adding a vial of peppermint oil to your list of diet aids. A study at Wheeling Jesuit University in West Virginia found that people who sniffed peppermint periodically throughout the day ate 2,800 fewer calories throughout the week. Focusing on the scent drives your attention away from cravings, says psychologist and lead researcher Bryan Raudenbush, Ph.D.

BREAKFAST

Hunger Level

FOOD/AMOUNT _____

_____

_____

_____

_____

_____

EMOTIONS _____

_____

_____

_____

_____

LUNCH

Hunger Level

FOOD/AMOUNT _____

_____

_____

_____

_____

_____

_____

EMOTIONS _____

_____

_____

_____

_____

DINNER

Hunger Level

FOOD/AMOUNT _____

_____

_____

_____

_____

_____

_____

EMOTIONS _____

_____

_____

_____

_____

SNACK 1

Hunger Level

TIME/PLACE _____

FOOD/AMOUNT _____

_____

EMOTIONS _____

_____

SNACK 2

Hunger Level

TIME/PLACE _____

FOOD/AMOUNT _____

_____

_____

EMOTIONS _____

_____

UNPLANNED EATING

Hunger Level

FOOD/AMOUNT _____

_____

_____

_____

TIME/PLACE _____

_____

_____

EMOTIONS _____

_____

_____

_____

_____

_____

_____

_____

DAILY MOVEMENT

Type of Activity	Minutes/Amount	How It Felt
AEROBIC Exercises:		
STRENGTHENING Exercises:		
FLEXIBILITY Exercises:		
BALANCE Exercises:		
INCIDENTAL MOVEMENT		

Weight-Loss Booster

Easy Calorie Trimmers Make one of these deletions from a meal and you'll save 100 calories.

- 2½ slices bacon from breakfast
- ½ cup brown rice from a stir-fry dinner
- 1 Tbsp. butter from a baked potato at dinner
- 1 Tbsp. peanut butter from a sandwich at lunch

DAILY ASSESSMENT

- What was your stress level today? If it was high, is there something you can do to alleviate it for tomorrow?

_____

_____

- Did you schedule in exercise and follow through? If not, what changed your plans?

_____

_____

- Did you discover anything about food/movement/yourself today that you found helpful or motivating?

_____

_____

- What nice thing did you do for yourself today?

_____

_____

- Final thoughts on the day: Are you pleased with how the day went? What went well? What do you resolve to change tomorrow?

_____

_____

_____

_____

_____

| **✻ DON'T FORGET** | _Check your to-do list before signing off for the night! It'll help you be ready for tomorrow._ |

How Was Your Week?

One key to successful weight loss is avoiding danger zones—locations where your willpower can easily give out. Maybe it's a colleague's desk, where a candy bowl dares you to indulge. Or your regular Friday night happy hour where you can't resist the bar chips and peanuts—they're part of the experience! Did any similar situations crop up this week, or do you anticipate any in the future? Jot down ways to circumvent temptation, either by avoiding the danger zone altogether or by using damage-control measures (having an apple ready so you can resist your colleague's candy, bringing your own snack with you to happy hour).

_____

_____

_____

_____

_____

_____

_____

_____

_____

_____

_____

GOALS FOR NEXT WEEK

_____

_____

_____

_____

_____

_____

_____

WEEK 7

WEEK 7

DAY 1

Breakfast: Breakfast Pizza
Lunch: Cheesy Chili
Snack 1: Movie Mix
Dinner: Healthy-Makeover Meatloaf
Snack 2: Pineapple Plate

DAY 2

Breakfast: Ham & Veggie Hash
Lunch: Sushi to Go
Snack 1: PB & J–Inspired Yogurt
Dinner: Ziti with Peas,
Grape Tomatoes & Ricotta
Snack 2: Cheese Bite

DAY 3

Breakfast: Banana–Peanut
Butter Smoothie
Lunch: Mexican Meal in Minutes
Snack 1: Strawberry Bagel Thin
Dinner: Turkey-Feta Burgers
Snack 2: Pudding Parfait

DAY 4

Breakfast: Strawberry Cereal
Lunch: Asian Chicken Salad
Snack 1: Iced-Coffee Break
Dinner: Almond-Crusted Tilapia
Snack 2: Hummus & Veggie Strips

DAY 5

Breakfast: California Breakfast
Bruschetta
Lunch: Mediterranean Hummus "Pizza"
Snack 1: Blueberry Lassi
Dinner: Chicken & Veggie Stir-Fry
Snack 2: Chips & Cheese

DAY 6

Breakfast: Sweet Stuffed Waffle
Lunch: Southwest Chicken Wraps
Snack 1: Cantaloupe Boat
Dinner: Spice-Rubbed Pork Tenderloin
Snack 2: Cocoa Fix

DAY 7

Breakfast: Peach Melba Yogurt
Lunch: Finger Food
Snack 1: Edamame Munchie
Dinner: Seared Salmon with
Sweet Potatoes
Snack 2: Prosciutto & Mozzarella Plate

Shopping List

For breakfasts, lunches, and dinners serving anywhere from one to six. Check recipes to make adjustments depending on the number of people you are feeding.

FRESH PRODUCE

12 tablespoons basil leaves
1 tablespoon chives
⅓ cup cilantro leaves
½ cup mint leaves
⅔ cup flat-leaf parsley leaves
5 green onions
1 pint (12 ounces) grape tomatoes
3 regular tomatoes
1 head Boston lettuce
½ small head napa (Chinese) cabbage
2 cups chopped romaine lettuce
1 bag (5 to 6 ounces) baby spinach
2 cups shredded carrots
4 stalks celery
2½ pounds green beans
1 package (10 ounces) sliced white mushrooms
2 medium and 1 large red bell pepper
1 large yellow bell pepper
6 medium red potatoes (1½ pounds total)
1 pound sweet potatoes
1 bunch radishes
1 small yellow summer squash
1 avocado
1 banana
1 pint (12 ounces) blackberries
1 small cantaloupe
20 grapes
2 small and 1 large orange
1 peach
1 pear
1 cup pineapple chunks
¼ cup pomegranate seeds
⅓ cup raspberries
1 pound strawberries

SEAFOOD

4 pieces skinless center-cut salmon fillets (1¼ pounds total)
4 tilapia fillets (1½ pounds total)

MEAT & POULTRY

2½ pounds skinless, boneless chicken-breast halves
1 pound ground chicken-breast or turkey-breast meat
1 pound pork tenderloin
3 pounds lean ground turkey
4 ounces thick-sliced ham or 4-ounce piece of ham
½ ounce very thinly sliced prosciutto

DAIRY

5 tablespoons shredded reduced-fat Cheddar or Monterey Jack cheese
1 wedge Laughing Cow ⅓ Less Fat Classic Cream Cheese Spread
1½ ounces reduced-fat feta cheese
1 ounce part-skim mozzarella cheese
1 stick part-skim mozzarella string cheese
1 cup low-fat (1%), low-sodium cottage cheese
1 container (6 ounces) sugar-free vanilla pudding

GRAIN PRODUCTS

¼ cup whole wheat orzo pasta
14 ounces whole-grain ziti pasta
2 packages (8.8 ounces each) precooked or Uncle Ben's Ready Rice brown rice

CANNED GOODS

1 can (15 ounces) pinto beans

FROZEN

- 2 Van's 8 Whole Grains waffles
- 7 Applegate Farms chicken nuggets
- ¼ cup frozen blueberries
- 24 ounces shelled edamame
- 2 cups frozen peas

MISCELLANEOUS

- 24 Emerald Cocoa Roast Almonds (dark-chocolate flavor) or Planters Smoked Almonds
- 1½ tablespoons bean dip
- 1 pouch (7½ ounces) Tabatchnick Vegetarian Chili
- 3 tablespoons Wholly Guacamole All Natural Classic Guacamole
- ⅔ cup hummus
- 1 cup Edy's/Dreyer's Slow Churned No Sugar Added Ice Cream, vanilla or Neapolitan flavor
- 1 cup Good Health Half Naked Popcorn
- 10 Food Should Taste Good Multigrain or Blue Corn tortilla chips
- 16 baked tortilla chips
- 1 Healthy Choice Chicken Tortilla microwavable soup bowl
- 1 cup Imagine Creamy Portobello Mushroom Soup
- 1 (6-piece) California maki sushi roll (made with brown rice, if available)*
- 15 sweet potato chips

Buy the day you'll be eating it.

DAY 1

TO-DO LIST

- Reread your pledge.

- Assess your schedule for today. Is anything going to make it difficult to stick to your diet? Strategize to overcome obstacles.

- Put some formal exercise on today's calendar or think about ways you can move your body.

- Plan for tomorrow's meals tonight. What are you going to eat? Do you have everything you need? If you're brown-bagging tomorrow's lunch, save time by assembling what you can now.

- Pack your journal or make sure you have a pen and paper (or a smartphone) for making notes throughout the day.

- Remind yourself of the commitment you made—and of how great you're going to feel as you make progress.

STICK-TO-IT STRATEGY

Moving On Hiccups in your new routine are bound to happen. If you get upset, you may punish yourself for transgressions by giving up because you've already messed up, and it can become a vicious cycle. Instead, follow the advice of philosopher-historian Will Durant: "Forget past mistakes. Forget failures. Forget everything except what you are going to do now and do it."

BREAKFAST

Hunger Level

FOOD/AMOUNT _____

_____

_____

_____

_____

EMOTIONS _____

_____

_____

_____

_____

_____

LUNCH

Hunger Level

FOOD/AMOUNT _____

_____

_____

_____

_____

EMOTIONS _____

_____

_____

_____

_____

TESTER TIP

"The fourth Sunday of each month, my church collects an offering for local food banks. Today, I proudly gave $15.87—the amount I saved after 15 days of no McDonald's sweet iced tea!"

—Jeanne Fishwick, 8 pounds and 2¾ inches lost

DINNER

Hunger Level

FOOD/AMOUNT _____

_____

_____

_____

_____

EMOTIONS _____

_____

_____

_____

_____

SNACK 1

Hunger Level

TIME/PLACE _____

FOOD/AMOUNT _____

EMOTIONS _____

SNACK 2

Hunger Level

TIME/PLACE _____

FOOD/AMOUNT _____

EMOTIONS _____

UNPLANNED EATING

Hunger Level

FOOD/AMOUNT _____

TIME/PLACE _____

EMOTIONS _____

DAILY MOVEMENT

Type of Activity	Minutes/Amount	How It Felt
AEROBIC Exercises:		
STRENGTHENING Exercises:		
FLEXIBILITY Exercises:		
BALANCE Exercises:		
INCIDENTAL MOVEMENT		

Hit the Pause Button You're on the verge of eating to soothe your sorrow, or anger, or stress, or loneliness. Whatever it is, pause. Tell yourself you'll take five minutes to do something else and see if you can let the desire to indulge pass. Call a friend, take your dog (or just yourself) for a walk, read a magazine, pull out your knitting, slip an exercise video into your DVD player, or pull out this workbook and write. Breaks that don't involve chewing may help you change direction and forgo that bowl of ice cream.

DAILY ASSESSMENT

● Losing weight and adhering to a meal plan can bring about changes beyond the number you see on the scale. Now that you're in Week 7, are there other aspects of your life that feel different? What are some ways that you can keep those feelings intact?

_____

● Today, what practices felt like they'd become healthy new habits? What still felt challenging?

_____

● Did you schedule in exercise and stick with it? If not, what changed your plans?

_____

● Did you discover anything about food/movement/yourself today that you found helpful or motivating?

_____

● What nice thing did you do for yourself today?

_____

● Final thoughts on the day: Are you pleased with how the day went? What went well? What do you resolve to change tomorrow?

_____

_____

_____

_____

_____

✳ **DON'T FORGET** | _Check your to-do list before signing off for the night! It'll help you be ready for tomorrow._

TO-DO LIST

- Assess your schedule for today. Is anything going to make it difficult to stick to your diet? Strategize to overcome obstacles.

- Put some formal exercise on today's calendar or think about extra ways you can move your body.

- Plan for tomorrow's meals tonight. What are you going to eat? Do you have everything you need? If you're brown-bagging tomorrow's lunch, save time by assembling what you can now.

- Pack your journal or make sure you have a pen and paper (or a smartphone) for making notes throughout the day.

- Remind yourself of the commitment you made—and of how great you're going to feel as you make progress.

MOVE MORE, LOSE MORE

Go the Extra Mile • If you commute using public transportation, get off the subway or bus a stop or two before your destination. If you take the train, board the car that will make you walk the farthest. • When you have to stand around and wait, pace back and forth. • Use the restroom one flight up from where you are (and take the stairs to get there). • Get more active with family and friends. Go to a museum, start a bowling league, or ride bikes.

BREAKFAST

Hunger Level

FOOD/AMOUNT _____

EMOTIONS _____

LUNCH

Hunger Level

FOOD/AMOUNT _____

_____

_____

_____

_____

_____

_____

EMOTIONS _____

_____

_____

_____

_____

_____

DINNER

Hunger Level

FOOD/AMOUNT _____

_____

_____

_____

_____

_____

_____

EMOTIONS _____

_____

_____

_____

_____

SNACK 1

Hunger Level

TIME/PLACE _____

FOOD/AMOUNT _____

EMOTIONS _____

UNPLANNED EATING

Hunger Level

FOOD/AMOUNT _____

TIME/PLACE _____

EMOTIONS _____

SNACK 2

Hunger Level

TIME/PLACE _____

FOOD/AMOUNT _____

EMOTIONS _____

DAILY MOVEMENT

Type of Activity	Minutes/Amount	How It Felt
AEROBIC Exercises:		
STRENGTHENING Exercises:		
FLEXIBILITY Exercises:		
BALANCE Exercises:		
INCIDENTAL MOVEMENT		

Once-a-Week Sweets Craving a cookie? Here are a few treats approved by Sam Cassetty, GHRI nutrition director. You can substitute one for a snack just one time a week. No seconds!

- 100% Whole Grain Fig Newtons (2 cookies)
- Back to Nature Apple Cinnamon Oat Grahams (2 full sheets), Golden Honey Oat Grahams (2 full sheets), or Crispy Oatmeal Cookies (2 cookies)
- Barbara's Bakery Snackimals in Wheat Free Oatmeal (about 10 cookies)
- Kashi Cookies (1 cookie) in Chocolate Almond Butter, Oatmeal Raisin Flax, or Oatmeal Dark Chocolate

DAILY ASSESSMENT

- Today, what practices felt like they'd become healthy new habits? What still felt challenging?

- Did you schedule in exercise and stick with it? If not, what changed your plans?

- Did you discover anything about food/movement/yourself today that you found helpful or motivating?

- What nice thing did you do for yourself today?

- Final thoughts on the day: Are you pleased with how the day went? What went well? What do you resolve to improve tomorrow?

✳ **DON'T FORGET** | *Check your to-do list before signing off for the night! It'll help you be ready for tomorrow.*

DAY 3

TO-DO LIST

- Assess your schedule for today. Is anything going to make it difficult to stick to your diet? Strategize to overcome obstacles.

- Put some formal exercise on today's calendar or think about extra ways you can move your body.

- Plan for tomorrow's meals tonight. What are you going to eat? Do you have everything you need? If you're brown-bagging tomorrow's lunch, save time by assembling what you can now.

- Pack your journal or make sure you have a pen and paper (or a smartphone) for making notes throughout the day.

- Remind yourself of the commitment you made—and of how great you're going to feel as you make progress.

ANTI-AGING EATING

The Spice Is Right It's not only foods—primarily fruits, vegetables, and grains—that confer antioxidant benefits; herbs and spices help fight aging, too. Among them, cinnamon is a standout: On its own, it's associated with a lower risk of heart attack, stroke, and type 2 diabetes. Sprinkle it on whole-grain cereal or toast, and it will boost that food's antioxidant content as well. Now *that's* sweet.

BREAKFAST

Hunger Level

FOOD/AMOUNT _____

EMOTIONS _____

LUNCH

*Hunger
Level*

FOOD/AMOUNT _____

_____
_____
_____
_____
_____
_____
_____

EMOTIONS _____

_____
_____
_____
_____
_____

DINNER

*Hunger
Level*

FOOD/AMOUNT _____

_____
_____
_____
_____
_____
_____

EMOTIONS _____

_____
_____
_____
_____
_____

SNACK 1

Hunger Level

TIME/PLACE _____

FOOD/AMOUNT _____

EMOTIONS _____

SNACK 2

Hunger Level

TIME/PLACE _____

FOOD/AMOUNT _____

EMOTIONS _____

UNPLANNED EATING

Hunger Level

FOOD/AMOUNT _____

TIME/PLACE _____

EMOTIONS _____

DAILY MOVEMENT

Type of Activity	Minutes/Amount	How It Felt
AEROBIC Exercises:		
STRENGTHENING Exercises:		
FLEXIBILITY Exercises:		
BALANCE Exercises:		
INCIDENTAL MOVEMENT		

Out-of-the-Box Breakfast "No time"—it's the classic rationalization for grabbing a donut off the pastry cart or pulling into the drive-through for a greasy egg sandwich. But who said your morning meal has to be a traditional breakfast food? If you think differently, there are plenty of healthy, if unconventional, options you can eat on the run. Here are three:

> **Energy Edibles** Munch on 1/3 cup trail mix (raisins, nuts, sunflower seeds) and sip 1 prepared packet of instant diet hot chocolate. *About 246 calories*

> **Sweet and Salty** Spread 6 reduced-fat Triscuits with 1½ tablespoons almond butter. Have with 1 tangerine or clementine. *About 314 calories*

> **Crunchy Fruit Creation** Stir 1 small handful of almonds (whole or sliced) into a single-serving cup of fruit in its own juice. *About 241 calories*

DAILY ASSESSMENT

- Today, what practices felt like they'd become healthy new habits? What still felt challenging?

- Did you schedule in exercise and stick with it? If not, what changed your plans?

- Did you discover anything about food/movement/yourself today that you found helpful or motivating?

- What nice thing did you do for yourself today?

- Final thoughts on the day: Are you pleased with how the day went? What went well? What do you resolve to improve tomorrow?

✱ DON'T FORGET | *Check your to-do list before signing off for the night! It'll help you be ready for tomorrow.*

DAY 4

TO-DO LIST

- Assess your schedule for today. Is anything going to make it difficult to stick to your diet? Strategize to overcome obstacles.

- Put some formal exercise on today's calendar or think about extra ways you can move your body.

- Plan for tomorrow's meals tonight. What are you going to eat? Do you have everything you need? If you're brown-bagging tomorrow's lunch, save time by assembling what you can now.

- Pack your journal or make sure you have a pen and paper (or a smartphone) for making notes throughout the day.

- Remind yourself of the commitment you made—and of how great you're going to feel as you make progress.

MOVE MORE, LOSE MORE

Avoid a Long Break If you just worked out several days in a row, pat yourself on the back. Don't, however, reward yourself with a comparable layoff. While exercise has immediate health benefits, like lowering blood pressure and improving blood sugar, animal research suggests that the effects wear off within days. Try to exercise every day or at least every other day.

BREAKFAST

Hunger Level

FOOD/AMOUNT

EMOTIONS

LUNCH

Hunger Level

FOOD/AMOUNT _____

_____

_____

_____

_____

_____

_____

EMOTIONS _____

_____

_____

_____

_____

_____

DINNER

Hunger Level

FOOD/AMOUNT _____

_____

_____

_____

_____

_____

_____

EMOTIONS _____

_____

_____

_____

_____

_____

SNACK 1

Hunger Level

TIME/PLACE _____

FOOD/AMOUNT _____

EMOTIONS _____

SNACK 2

Hunger Level

TIME/PLACE _____

FOOD/AMOUNT _____

EMOTIONS _____

UNPLANNED EATING

Hunger Level

FOOD/AMOUNT _____

TIME/PLACE _____

EMOTIONS _____

DAILY MOVEMENT

Type of Activity	Minutes/Amount	How It Felt
AEROBIC Exercises:		
STRENGTHENING Exercises:		
FLEXIBILITY Exercises:		
BALANCE Exercises:		
INCIDENTAL MOVEMENT		

Break Your Fast! It's well known that people who bypass breakfast tend to compensate by loading up on calories later in the day. But research suggests that meal-skipping also contributes to poorer food choices. In one study, Cornell University researchers had 128 students fast for 18 hours (eating nothing after 6 P.M.), then invited them to lunch multiple times over 12 days. At lunch, students who hadn't eaten breakfast were more likely to choose starchy, high-calorie foods over nutrient-dense vegetable dishes.

DAILY ASSESSMENT

⬤ Today, what practices felt like they'd become healthy new habits? What still felt challenging?

_____

_____

⬤ Did you schedule in exercise and stick with it? If not, what changed your plans?

_____

_____

⬤ Did you discover anything about food/movement/yourself today that you found helpful or motivating?

_____

_____

⬤ What nice thing did you do for yourself today?

_____

_____

⬤ Final thoughts on the day: Are you pleased with how the day went? What went well? What do you resolve to improve tomorrow?

_____

_____

_____

_____

_____

_____

✱ **DON'T FORGET** | _Check your to-do list before signing off for the night! It'll help you be ready for tomorrow._

TO-DO LIST

- Assess your schedule for today. Is anything going to make it difficult to stick to your diet? Strategize to overcome obstacles.

- Put some formal exercise on today's calendar or think about extra ways you can move your body.

- Plan for tomorrow's meals tonight. What are you going to eat? Do you have everything you need? If you're brown-bagging tomorrow's lunch, save time by assembling what you can now.

- Pack your journal or make sure you have a pen and paper (or a smartphone) for making notes throughout the day.

- Remind yourself of the commitment you made—and of how great you're going to feel as you make progress.

MORE MINDFUL EATING

Breathing Away Temptation If you're tempted to raid the refrigerator to make up for a bad day, try this: Place your hands on your belly and inhale slowly through your nose, letting the air fill your belly. Count to five as you inhale, then exhale (also through your nose) on the same count. Focus on the rise and fall of your belly. Repeat. Calming, focused breathing can help you walk away from the fridge.

BREAKFAST

Hunger Level

FOOD/AMOUNT _____

_____

_____

_____

_____

EMOTIONS _____

_____

_____

_____

_____

LUNCH

Hunger Level

FOOD/AMOUNT _____

_____

_____

_____

_____

EMOTIONS _____

_____

_____

_____

_____

=== TESTER TIP ===

"Two things I really rely on are my kitchen scale—to double-check my portions—and an online calorie counter."

—Carol Scudder-Danilowicz, 8½ pounds and 4¾ inches lost

DINNER

Hunger Level

FOOD/AMOUNT _____

_____

_____

_____

_____

EMOTIONS _____

_____

_____

_____

_____

SNACK 1

Hunger Level

TIME/PLACE _____

FOOD/AMOUNT _____

EMOTIONS _____

SNACK 2

Hunger Level

TIME/PLACE _____

FOOD/AMOUNT _____

EMOTIONS _____

UNPLANNED EATING

Hunger Level

FOOD/AMOUNT _____

TIME/PLACE _____

EMOTIONS _____

DAILY MOVEMENT

Type of Activity	Minutes/Amount	How It Felt
AEROBIC Exercises:		
STRENGTHENING Exercises:		
FLEXIBILITY Exercises:		
BALANCE Exercises:		
INCIDENTAL MOVEMENT		

Portion Sizes at a Glance Overly generous helpings can cause weight regain. As you go forward into weight maintenance, don't forget what constitutes a proper portion size. You don't have to weigh and/or measure everything. Here's a cheat sheet to help you eyeball foods:

- **3 ounces of fish, poultry, or meat = a smartphone**
- **1 ounce of cheese = four dice**
- **2 tablespoons of dressing = a shot glass**
- **$1/2$ cup of grains, rice, or pasta = a tennis ball**
- **A small dinner roll = a computer mouse**
- **$1/4$ cup of nuts = a large egg**
- **1 teaspoon of butter = a Scrabble tile**

DAILY ASSESSMENT

- Today, what practices felt like they'd become healthy new habits? What still felt challenging?

_____

- Did you schedule in exercise and stick with it? If not, what changed your plans?

_____

- Did you discover anything about food/movement/yourself today that you found helpful or motivating?

_____

- What nice thing did you do for yourself today?

_____

- Final thoughts on the day: Are you pleased with how the day went? What went well? What do you resolve to improve tomorrow?

_____
_____
_____
_____
_____

| ✳ **DON'T FORGET** | _Check your to-do list before signing off for the night! It'll help you be ready for tomorrow._ |

DAY 6

TO-DO LIST

- Assess your schedule for today. Is anything going to make it difficult to stick to your diet? Strategize to overcome obstacles.

- Put some formal exercise on today's calendar or think about extra ways you can move your body.

- Plan for tomorrow's meals tonight. What are you going to eat? Do you have everything you need? If you're brown-bagging tomorrow's lunch, save time by assembling what you can now.

- Pack your journal or make sure you have a pen and paper (or a smartphone) for making notes throughout the day.

- Remind yourself of the commitment you made—and of how great you're going to feel as you make progress.

ANTI-AGING EATING

Coffee or Tea? Once a dietary villain, coffee has been associated with a lower risk of type 2 diabetes, melanoma, and Parkinson's disease. Moderate coffee drinkers may have better memories and appear to be less likely to die from heart disease. And tea has its perks: Two cups a day can help strengthen your immune system, fight cancer, protect tooth enamel, and prevent memory loss.

BREAKFAST

Hunger Level

FOOD/AMOUNT _____

_____

_____

_____

_____

_____

EMOTIONS _____

_____

_____

_____

LUNCH

*Hunger
Level*

FOOD/AMOUNT _____

_____
_____
_____
_____
_____
_____

EMOTIONS _____

_____
_____
_____
_____
_____

DINNER

*Hunger
Level*

FOOD/AMOUNT _____

_____
_____
_____
_____
_____
_____

EMOTIONS _____

_____
_____
_____
_____
_____

SNACK 1

Hunger Level

TIME/PLACE _____

FOOD/AMOUNT _____

EMOTIONS _____

SNACK 2

Hunger Level

TIME/PLACE _____

FOOD/AMOUNT _____

EMOTIONS _____

UNPLANNED EATING

Hunger Level

FOOD/AMOUNT _____

TIME/PLACE _____

EMOTIONS _____

DAILY MOVEMENT

Type of Activity	Minutes/Amount	How It Felt
AEROBIC Exercises:		
STRENGTHENING Exercises:		
FLEXIBILITY Exercises:		
BALANCE Exercises:		
INCIDENTAL MOVEMENT		

Fitness, Family-Style Think of physical activity not as exercise, but as family time. Here's a list of things you can do together:

Hike	Bowl	Go apple- or berry-picking
Bike	Play miniature golf	Play touch football
Rock/wall-climb	Play Ping-Pong	Ice skate
Canoe, kayak, row, do stand-up paddling	Take a martial arts class	Walk the dog

DAILY ASSESSMENT

- Today, what practices felt like they'd become healthy new habits? What still felt challenging?

_____

_____

- Did you schedule in exercise and stick with it? If not, what changed your plans?

_____

_____

- Did you discover anything about food/movement/yourself today that you found helpful or motivating?

_____

_____

- What nice thing did you do for yourself today?

_____

_____

- Final thoughts on the day: Are you pleased with how the day went? What went well? What do you resolve to improve tomorrow?

_____

_____

_____

_____

_____

_____

* DON'T FORGET | *Check your to-do list before signing off for the night! It'll help you be ready for tomorrow.*

DAY 7

TO-DO LIST

- Assess your schedule for today. Is anything going to make it difficult to stick to your diet? Strategize to overcome obstacles.

- Put some formal exercise on today's calendar or think about extra ways you can move your body.

- Plan for tomorrow's meals tonight. What are you going to eat? Do you have everything you need? If you're brown-bagging tomorrow's lunch, save time by assembling what you can now.

- Pack your journal or make sure you have a pen and paper (or a smartphone) for making notes throughout the day.

- Remind yourself of the commitment you made—and congratulate yourself for all your progress!

CRAVINGS CONTROL

Higher Contrast, Lower Calories When Cornell researchers randomly gave partygoers red or white plates, then instructed them to serve themselves from a buffet of pasta, those who had a low-contrast meal (e.g., white-Alfredo-sauced pasta on a white plate) ended up serving themselves 22% more than those who chose the high-contrast meal (e.g., red-tomato-sauced pasta on a white plate).

BREAKFAST

Hunger Level

FOOD/AMOUNT

EMOTIONS

LUNCH

Hunger Level

FOOD/AMOUNT _____

_____

_____

_____

_____

_____

_____

EMOTIONS _____

_____

_____

_____

_____

_____

DINNER

Hunger Level

FOOD/AMOUNT _____

_____

_____

_____

_____

_____

_____

EMOTIONS _____

_____

_____

_____

_____

_____

SNACK 1

Hunger
Level

TIME/PLACE _____

_____

FOOD/AMOUNT _____

_____

EMOTIONS _____

_____

SNACK 2

Hunger
Level

TIME/PLACE _____

_____

FOOD/AMOUNT _____

_____

EMOTIONS _____

_____

UNPLANNED EATING

Hunger
Level

FOOD/AMOUNT _____

_____

_____

_____

TIME/PLACE _____

_____

_____

EMOTIONS _____

_____

_____

_____

_____

_____

_____

DAILY MOVEMENT

Type of Activity	Minutes/Amount	How It Felt
AEROBIC Exercises:		
STRENGTHENING Exercises:		
FLEXIBILITY Exercises:		
BALANCE Exercises:		
INCIDENTAL MOVEMENT		

Diet-Friendly Drinks The innovative cocktail trend is so widespread and enticing, it could make a teetotaler think twice. While alcohol has its place in a healthy diet—both women and men can enjoy a drink per day on the 7 *Years Younger Anti-Aging Breakthrough Diet*—the calories can add up. Here are four of the lowest-calorie cocktail picks; be sure to pay attention to portion sizes:

- **Mimosa (4 ounces):** *80 calories*
- **Bloody Mary (5 ounces):** *120 calories*
- **Wine (red or white, 5 ounces):** *120 calories*
- **Green-apple martini (3 ounces):** *150 calories*
- **Manhattan (2½ ounces):** *120 calories*

DAILY ASSESSMENT

- Today, what practices felt like they'd become healthy new habits? What still felt challenging?

- Did you schedule in exercise and stick with it? If not, what changed your plans?

- Did you discover anything about food/movement/yourself today that you found helpful or motivating?

- What nice thing did you do for yourself today?

- Final thoughts on the day: Are you pleased with how the day went? What went well? What do you resolve to improve tomorrow?

How Did You Do?

Congratulations! It takes willpower and stamina to change habits. You deserve praise for the work you've put in over the past seven weeks.

Now is a good time to look at your results, celebrate your successes, and make plans for continuing this healthy new lifestyle into the future.

To begin, what are the results of your diet? Record them here. Then write about how you feel. Are you pleased with your results? Summarize your eating and exercise habits now. Are they markedly different than when you first began 7 *Years Younger: The Anti-Aging Breakthrough Diet*? What, if anything, do you still need to work on? What are your goals for the future? What strategies can you employ to make sure the pounds don't come back?

WEIGHT LOST _____

_____

_____

_____

_____

**DESCRIBE YOUR RESULTS
AND CHANGES THAT YOU'VE MADE** _____

_____

_____

_____

_____

_____

_____

_____

_____

_____

_____

_____

You've essentially just written your own personal diet book! All the information, actions, and emotions you've chronicled in this workbook will help you stay motivated in the future and serve as a reminder of just how far you've come. As you move into maintenance mode, you'll have everything you need for continued success.

The eating plan in 7 *Years Younger: The Anti-Aging Breakthrough Diet* wasn't just a weight-loss road map for seven weeks; it's a template for a new way of living. You can continue to follow it to the letter to help you keep on losing—or, if you've reached your ideal weight, recalibrate the calories a little to stay there. One way to calculate a maintenance calorie level is based on your ideal weight: It takes about 15 calories a day to support one pound, so if your ideal weight is 140 pounds, you should be eating 2,100 calories a day to sustain it. (That's based on 140 x 15 = 2,100.)

However, keep in mind that this formula only approximates your optimal calorie intake—there are a lot of variables. If you aren't active, for instance, you could gain weight at 2,100 calories a day. If you walk or jog five miles a day, you may need more calories. Use the formula to give yourself a starting point; then monitor your weight on the scale. Weigh yourself daily, or at least two to three times a week. A fluctuation of three pounds from one day to the next is normal. But hitting five pounds above where you want to be is an indication that you've set your calorie count too high—or that you're straying from the goals you've set. If this happens, think about what you've been eating over the last few weeks. Return to the Jumpstart (Week 1) and begin a new food diary to help you get back to where you want to be. Stay physically active, too: Research shows that this is critical for maintaining weight loss—and it's the best thing you can do to continue fighting aging, too.

As time goes on, hold on to the feeling you've had for the last seven weeks. Being in control of your health and feeling lighter, leaner, and younger—that's going to be your best maintenance tool of all!

COVER DESIGN BY Jill Armus
BOOK DESIGN BY Peter Hemmel
COVER IMAGE Vladyslav Starozhylov/Shutterstock.com

ISBN 978-1-936297-27-6

10 9 8 7 6 5 4 3 2 1

PUBLISHED BY
Hearst Magazines
300 West 57th Street
New York, NY 10019

Good Housekeeping is a registered trademark and 7YY is a trademark of Hearst Communications, Inc.
www.goodhousekeeping.com
www.7yearsyounger.com
DISTRIBUTED TO THE TRADE BY Hachette Book Group

All US and Canadian orders:
Hachette Book Group
Order Department
Three Center Plaza
Boston, MA 02108
CALL TOLL FREE 1-800-759-0190
FAX TOLL FREE 1-800-286-9471

For information regarding discounts to corporations, organizations, non-book retailers and wholesalers; mail order catalogs; and premiums, contact:
Special Markets Department
Hachette Book Group
237 Park Avenue
New York, NY 10017
CALL TOLL FREE 1-800-222-6747
FAX TOLL FREE 1-800-222-6902

For all international orders:
Hachette Book Group
237 Park Avenue
New York, NY 10017
TEL 212-364-1325
FAX 800-364-0933
international@hbgusa.com

PRINTED IN THE USA